## 30 Day Cholesterol Program

### Some Basic Life Extending Facts

The link between high-cholesterol levels and coronary heart disease (CHD) is overwhelming; the higher the cholesterol level, the higher the risk of CHD.

**Cholesterol is not static;** it changes as we age or alter our lifestyles. It *can* therefore be lowered.

**Knowing your cholesterol level is vital.** Everyone aged 20 and up should have their cholesterol checked every second year till the age of 40. It the level is below 200, test every five years. If cholesterol level is over 200, again retest every year.

**Get your blood lipid profile and maintain a proper balance** of low levels of VLDLs (very low-density lipoproteins) and LDLs (low-density lipoproteins), and high levels of HDLs (high-density lipoproteins). It is important to keep LDL cholesterol, which is an independent risk factor, below 130 mg/dl and your HDL above 35 mg/dl.

There is evidence that polyunsaturated fats (safflower, sunflower, corn, soybean and cotton seed oils) help reduce overall cholesterol without lowering your HDLs. So do monounsaturated fats like oil from olives, peanuts and avocados.

**If you're still eating a lot of** eggs, red meat, ice cream, cream, whole milk, and butter, you should be able to get a noticeable lowering by switching to skim milk, low-fat dairy products, margerine and fish, and cutting back sharply on eggs and meat.

Adding foods like oat bran, corn bran, rice bran, beans and rice could help as well.

**Regular exercise is important.** It helps increase your HDLs; a reduced HDL cholesterol level is a major risk factor.

**Keeping your weight under control,** sticking to low fat, high fiber diet and keeping blood lipids in a healthy balance is a lifelong effort. It is never too early to start. Start now. This book will help you lead a long and healthy life.

Health Care in
**Orient Paperbacks**

Mayo Clinic on Managing Diabetes (*Illus.*)
Mayo Clinic on Digestive Health (*Illus.*)
Mayo Clinic on Arthritis (*Illus.*)
Mayo Clinic on High Blood Pressure (*Illus.*)
The Dermatologist's Guide to Looking Younger

Overcoming Migraines & Other Headaches
Cure Aches and Pains through Osteopathy
Heart Disease and High Blood Pressure
Hot Water Therapy
Overcoming Stress

Preventing & Surviving Heart Attacks
Headaches: The Self-Help Book
Preventing Heart Disease: Exercising for a Healthy Heart
Antioxidants: Vitamins C & E for Health
Conquering Diabetes Naturally

Asthma in Children
Healthy Heart Diet Book

THE BARBARA KRAUS

# 30 DAY CHOLESTEROL PROGRAM

A Physician Approved Diet and
Exercise Plan for Lowering
Your Cholesterol

Orient Paperbacks
DELHI | MUMBAI | HYDERABAD

For Heart Patients
Throughout the World


**Acknowledgments**

Thank you to Adrienne Ingrum for making this project possible, and her assistant, Charles de Kay, for his gracious support. A very special thanks to Elza Dinwiddie-Boyd for lending her professional skills to the completion of the book.

ISBN 81-222-0136-9

1st Indian Edition 1992

*The Barbara Kraus 30-Day Cholesterol Program: A Diet and Exercise Plan for Lowering Your Cholesterol*





Cover design by Vision Studio

Published in arrangement with
The Putnam Publishing Group, Inc., New York

Published by
**Orient Paperbacks**
(A division of Vision Books Pvt. Ltd.)
Madarsa Road, Kashmere Gate, Delhi-110 006

Printed in India at
Kay Kay Printers, Delhi-110 007

Cover Printed at
Ravindra Printing Press, Delhi-110 006

# Preface

Elevated cholesterol forms an important risk factor for the development of atheroscelerosis which in turns leads to life threatening diseases such as coronary artery disease and cerebral vascular disease. Unlike some of the other risk factors, the redeeming feature here is that reduction of cholestrol can lead to dramatic decrease in the risk of coronary heart disease. Studies have shown that every 1 per cent reduction of total cholesterol leads to a 2 per cent reduction in the risk for coronary heart disease. Though many pharmacological agents are available now for the reduction of elevated cholesterol levels many of these are not only expensive but most have several side effects. It is, therefore, pertinent specially in the Indian context to look for methods that can effectively lower cholesterol without the use of pharmacological agents. Disciplined diet and regular exercise measures are known to be responsible for the major reduction in the incidence of coronary artery disease in many Western countries and similar results should be achievable in India and other countries of Asia, Middle East and Africa as well.

This book, *The Barbara Kraus 30-Day Cholesterol Program*, helps to introduce in a scientific manner the danger of increased cholesterol and the importance of the need to decrease cholesterol levels. Risk factor analysis which is a great primer to the proper management of elevated cholesterol is thoroughly discussed in this book in simple and descriptive language. The dietary and exercise guidelines given in the book are also based on sound scientific principles and written in a manner that would make it understandable to even the uninitiated. In view of increasing incidence of coronary artery disease in our country in the past years, this book would be of immense use and help not only to those who suffer from high cholesterol but also for anybody who desires to lead a life free of debilititating illness such as coronary artery and cerebro-vascular diseases.

Prof. M. Khalilullah
Padma Shree, Padma Bhushan
MBBS, MD (Med), DM (Cardiology),
D.Sc (Med) Honoris Causa
Director, Professor & Head of Cardiology
Govind Ballabh Pant Hospital,
New Delhi

# Contents

# Foreword

This text, *The Barbara Kraus 30-Day Cholesterol Program*, is designed to help those individuals who need to lower their serum cholesterol levels and thereby decrease the risk for coronary heart disease. The author has carefully delineated the risk factors involved in its development. During the last decade, progress has been made in establishing the cholesterol/coronary heart disease hypothesis and in defining the role of an elevated serum cholesterol in the pathogenesis of atherosclerosis. Coronary heart disease is often a result of the deposit of cholesterol and calcium in one or more of the three major coronary vessels that supply the muscle mass of the heart. Despite increasing evidence of the dangers of abnormally elevated serum lipids and the value of lipid reduction therapy, recent studies indicate that high serum lipids have been neglected even in patients with known atherosclerosis.

The impact of the lack of treatment of atherosclerosis is extremely costly in terms of medical intervention such as coronary artery bypass grafting or coronary angioplasty (a procedure in which balloons are inserted into the coronary vessels to expand and improve the blood flow through these vessels). Therefore, to deal effectively with coronary heart disease, risk factor modification is the primary goal of the medical community.

Therapy for lipid disorders includes dietary changes, maintenance of ideal body weight, aerobic exercise, smoking cessation, anti-hypertension therapy, and the use of medication where required. In October of 1987 the National Cholesterol Education Program recommended that vigorous dietary measures be implemented for all individuals with elevated serum cholesterol totals. Proper nutritional advice remains the basic initial step for most, if not all, patients with lipoprotein abnormalities. Studies indicate that every 1-percent reduction of total cholesterol translates into a 2-percent reduction in the risk for coronary heart disease.

In general, specific dietary instruction and achievement of ideal body weight are the goals to be achieved. These goals require innovative and careful nutritional programs with regular follow-up and continued encouragement by an enthusiastic and confident nutritional staff.

All of the pharmacological agents used to lower abnormally elevated lipids are expensive and have major side effects. Despite the promising new drugs that are currently being developed or are available, strict, dedicated dietary management remains the cornerstone for the prevention of significant coronary artery disease. For many high-risk patients the goals of cholesterol lowering can be achieved by dietary therapy alone. It is important that dietary therapy not be prematurely regarded as a failure.

The materials in this text offer basic guidelines for successful intervention and management of high serum cholesterol. Risk factor analysis in the treatment and evaluation of patients with an elevated serum cholesterol is crucial to its proper management. The risk factors are thoroughly discussed in this text, but it has to be emphasized that male sex is a risk factor. The rate of coronary heart disease is three to four times higher in men in their middle years of life than in women and roughly twice as high in elderly men as in elderly women.

Although the incidence of coronary heart disease has decreased during the last decade because of dietary alterations, it still remains the major cause of death in Western society. Despite the lowering of the coronary heart disease mortality rates in the United States, it is clear that risk factor modification must be practiced with a greater degree of discipline by the general American public. As a nation we cannot afford to maintain our current unhealthy dietary and lifestyle habits and expect modern technology to bail us out once disease develops. The technology that is available for the improvement of blood flow to the heart muscle is expensive, and as with any interventional therapy, potentially risky for the patient. With the escalating cost of health care and with the limited allocation of health care resources, it is extremely important that a more basic approach be devised and implemented on a nationwide basis to further decrease the rate of development of coronary artery disease and thereby to lessen the incidence of sudden cardiac death and death by recurrent heart attacks. The book that you are about to read is a step in the right direction.

ALAN BECKLES, M.D.
Beth Israel Medical Center
New York, NY

# 1
# Elevated Cholesterol: The Implications

Although many knowledgeable people—doctors, nutritionists, health food advocates—have known for years about the dangers of high levels of serum cholesterol in the body, only recently has widespread attention been focused on the amount of saturated fat in our daily diets and the relationship of that consumption to the cholesterol levels found in our blood supply. The average American diet is far too high in saturated fats. A government study indicates that if all Americans reduced the cholesterol in their blood by 25 percent, coronary heart disease in this country would drop by 50 percent. You *can* lower your serum cholesterol to safe levels. By doing so, you decrease the risk of developing atherosclerosis, a major factor in coronary heart disease.

## *ATHEROSCLEROSIS, NOT ARTERIOSCLEROSIS*

Arteriosclerosis is the name for the general category of arterial disease; usually it refers to the hardening of the arteries found in the elderly. This hardening effect is said to be caused by calcium deposits. As a matter of fact, many experts believe that the narrowing effect of atherosclerosis is far more deadly than the hardening in arteriosclerosis.

Atherosclerosis is the name given to the condition of the artery walls when the network of connective tissue called plaque has formed, clogging and narrowing the passage through which the vital, life-giving, life-sustaining blood flows. Atherosclerotic plaque on artery walls causes angina and heart attacks. Excessive levels of cholesterol and triglycerides are implicated in the formation of arterial plaque. Atherosclerosis is categorized by irregularly distributed lipid deposits in the intima (the interior arterial lining) of large- and medium-sized arteries. Atherosclerosis may be an asymptomatic disease, one that gradually occurs without the knowledge of its victim. It may be a silent killer, much like hypertension.

The danger lies in the narrowing of the arteries. Your arteries can begin narrowing while you are very young. Youth is no safeguard against the deadly arterial lesions formed as a result of excessive consumption of cholesterol.

## *BLOOD LIPIDS: CHOLESTEROL AND TRIGLYCERIDES*

Just what is cholesterol and why is it so important? Cholesterol is an essential constituent of animal cells; without it the cells of all animals, humans too, will not function properly and the organism will die. This fatty substance known as cholesterol is a life-giving, life-sustaining force. As potent as it is to maintaining life—when it is in proper balance—it is equally threatening to life when it is out of balance. Too much cholesterol can be lethal. Coronary heart disease (CHD), a direct result of high levels of serum cholesterol, causes more deaths per year than all forms of cancer combined.

The blood fats (lipids) cholesterol and triglycerides are both found in the bloodstream, but they differ in chemical makeup.

that the narrowing effect of atherosclerosis is far more deadly than the hardening in arteriosclerosis.

Atherosclerosis is the name given to the condition of the artery walls when the network of connective tissue called plaque has formed, clogging and narrowing the passage through which the vital, life-giving, life-sustaining blood flows. Atherosclerotic plaque on artery walls causes angina and heart attacks. Excessive levels of cholesterol and triglycerides are implicated in the formation of arterial plaque. Atherosclerosis is categorized by irregularly distributed lipid deposits in the intima (the interior arterial lining) of large- and medium-sized arteries. Atherosclerosis may be an asymptomatic disease, one that gradually occurs without the knowledge of its victim. It may be a silent killer, much like hypertension.

The danger lies in the narrowing of the arteries. Your arteries can begin narrowing while you are very young. Youth is no safeguard against the deadly arterial lesions formed as a result of excessive consumption of cholesterol.

## *BLOOD LIPIDS: CHOLESTEROL AND TRIGLYCERIDES*

Just what is cholesterol and why is it so important? Cholesterol is an essential constituent of animal cells; without it the cells of all animals, humans too, will not function properly and the organism will die. This fatty substance known as cholesterol is a life-giving, life-sustaining force. As potent as it is to maintaining life—when it is in proper balance—it is equally threatening to life when it is out of balance. Too much cholesterol can be lethal. Coronary heart disease (CHD), a direct result of high levels of serum cholesterol, causes more deaths per year than all forms of cancer combined.

The blood fats (lipids) cholesterol and triglycerides are both found in the bloodstream, but they differ in chemical makeup.

# 1
# Elevated Cholesterol: The Implications

Although many knowledgeable people—doctors, nutritionists, health food advocates—have known for years about the dangers of high levels of serum cholesterol in the body, only recently has widespread attention been focused on the amount of saturated fat in our daily diets and the relationship of that consumption to the cholesterol levels found in our blood supply. The average American diet is far too high in saturated fats. A government study indicates that if all Americans reduced the cholesterol in their blood by 25 percent, coronary heart disease in this country would drop by 50 percent. You *can* lower your serum cholesterol to safe levels. By doing so, you decrease the risk of developing atherosclerosis, a major factor in coronary heart disease.

## *ATHEROSCLEROSIS*, *NOT ARTERIOSCLEROSIS*

Arteriosclerosis is the name for the general category of arterial disease; usually it refers to the hardening of the arteries found in the elderly. This hardening effect is said to be caused by calcium deposits. As a matter of fact, many experts believe

men in their middle years of life than in women and roughly twice as high in elderly men as in elderly women.

Although the incidence of coronary heart disease has decreased during the last decade because of dietary alterations, it still remains the major cause of death in Western society. Despite the lowering of the coronary heart disease mortality rates in the United States, it is clear that risk factor modification must be practiced with a greater degree of discipline by the general American public. As a nation we cannot afford to maintain our current unhealthy dietary and lifestyle habits and expect modern technology to bail us out once disease develops. The technology that is available for the improvement of blood flow to the heart muscle is expensive, and as with any interventional therapy, potentially risky for the patient. With the escalating cost of health care and with the limited allocation of health care resources, it is extremely important that a more basic approach be devised and implemented on a nationwide basis to further decrease the rate of development of coronary artery disease and thereby to lessen the incidence of sudden cardiac death and death by recurrent heart attacks. The book that you are about to read is a step in the right direction.

ALAN BECKLES, M.D.
Beth Israel Medical Center
New York, NY

factor modification is the primary goal of the medical community.

Therapy for lipid disorders includes dietary changes, maintenance of ideal body weight, aerobic exercise, smoking cessation, anti-hypertension therapy, and the use of medication where required. In October of 1987 the National Cholesterol Education Program recommended that vigorous dietary measures be implemented for all individuals with elevated serum cholesterol totals. Proper nutritional advice remains the basic initial step for most, if not all, patients with lipoprotein abnormalities. Studies indicate that every 1-percent reduction of total cholesterol translates into a 2-percent reduction in the risk for coronary heart disease.

In general, specific dietary instruction and achievement of ideal body weight are the goals to be achieved. These goals require innovative and careful nutritional programs with regular follow-up and continued encouragement by an enthusiastic and confident nutritional staff.

All of the pharmacological agents used to lower abnormally elevated lipids are expensive and have major side effects. Despite the promising new drugs that are currently being developed or are available, strict, dedicated dietary management remains the cornerstone for the prevention of significant coronary artery disease. For many high-risk patients the goals of cholesterol lowering can be achieved by dietary therapy alone. It is important that dietary therapy not be prematurely regarded as a failure.

The materials in this text offer basic guidelines for successful intervention and management of high serum cholesterol. Risk factor analysis in the treatment and evaluation of patients with an elevated serum cholesterol is crucial to its proper management. The risk factors are thoroughly discussed in this text, but it has to be emphasized that male sex is a risk factor. The rate of coronary heart disease is three to four times higher in

# Foreword

This text, *The Barbara Kraus 30-Day Cholesterol Program*, is designed to help those individuals who need to lower their serum cholesterol levels and thereby decrease the risk for coronary heart disease. The author has carefully delineated the risk factors involved in its development. During the last decade, progress has been made in establishing the cholesterol/coronary heart disease hypothesis and in defining the role of an elevated serum cholesterol in the pathogenesis of atherosclerosis. Coronary heart disease is often a result of the deposit of cholesterol and calcium in one or more of the three major coronary vessels that supply the muscle mass of the heart. Despite increasing evidence of the dangers of abnormally elevated serum lipids and the value of lipid reduction therapy, recent studies indicate that high serum lipids have been neglected even in patients with known atherosclerosis.

The impact of the lack of treatment of atherosclerosis is extremely costly in terms of medical intervention such as coronary artery bypass grafting or coronary angioplasty (a procedure in which balloons are inserted into the coronary vessels to expand and improve the blood flow through these vessels). Therefore, to deal effectively with coronary heart disease, risk

# Contents

need to decrease cholesterol levels. Risk factor analysis which is a great primer to the proper management of elevated cholesterol is thoroughly discussed in this book in simple and descriptive language. The dietary and exercise guidelines given in the book are also based on sound scientific principles and written in a manner that would make it understandable to even the uninitiated. In view of increasing incidence of coronary artery disease in our country in the past years, this book would be of immense use and help not only to those who suffer from high cholesterol but also for anybody who desires to lead a life free of debilititating illness such as coronary artery and cerebro-vascular diseases.

Prof. M. Khalilullah
Padma Shree, Padma Bhushan
MBBS, MD (Med), DM (Cardiology),
D.Sc (Med) Honoris Causa
Director, Professor & Head of Cardiology
Govind Ballabh Pant Hospital,
New Delhi

# Preface

Elevated cholesterol forms an important risk factor for the development of atheroscelerosis which in turns leads to life threatening diseases such as coronary artery disease and cerebral vascular disease. Unlike some of the other risk factors, the redeeming feature here is that reduction of cholestrol can lead to dramatic decrease in the risk of coronary heart disease. Studies have shown that every 1 per cent reduction of total cholesterol leads to a 2 per cent reduction in the risk for coronary heart disease. Though many pharmacological agents are available now for the reduction of elevated cholesterol levels many of these are not only expensive but most have several side effects. It is, therefore, pertinent specially in the Indian context to look for methods that can effectively lower cholesterol without the use of pharmacological agents. Disciplined diet and regular exercise measures are known to be responsible for the major reduction in the incidence of coronary artery disease in many Western countries and similar results should be achievable in India and other countries of Asia, Middle East and Africa as well.

This book, *The Barbara Kraus 30-Day Cholesterol Program*, helps to introduce in a scientific manner the danger of increased cholesterol and the importance of the

For Heart Patients
Throughout the World

**Acknowledgments**

Thank you to Adrienne Ingrum for making this project possible, and her assistant, Charles de Kay, for his gracious support. A very special thanks to Elza Dinwiddie-Boyd for lending her professional skills to the completion of the book.

ISBN 81-222-0136-9

1st Indian Edition 1992

*The Barbara Kraus 30-Day Cholesterol Program:*
*A Diet and Exercise Plan for Lowering Your Cholesterol*



Cover design by Vision Studio

Published in arrangement with
The Putnam Publishing Group, Inc., New York

Published by
**Orient Paperbacks**
(A division of Vision Books Pvt. Ltd.)
Madarsa Road, Kashmere Gate, Delhi-110 006

Printed in India at
Kay Kay Printers, Delhi-110 007

Cover Printed at
Ravindra Printing Press, Delhi-110 006

THE BARBARA KRAUS

# 30 DAY CHOLESTEROL PROGRAM

A Physician Approved Diet and Exercise Plan for Lowering Your Cholesterol

Orient Paperbacks
DELHI | MUMBAI | HYDERABAD

# 30 Day Cholesterol Program

## Some Basic Life Extending Facts

The link between high-cholesterol levels and coronary heart disease (CHD) is overwhelming; the higher the cholesterol level, the higher the risk of CHD.

**Cholesterol is not static;** it changes as we age or alter our lifestyles. It *can* therefore be lowered.

**Knowing your cholesterol level is vital.** Everyone aged 20 and up should have their cholesterol checked every second year till the age of 40. It the level is below 200, test every five years. If cholesterol level is over 200, again retest every year.

**Get your blood lipid profile and maintain a proper balance** of low levels of VLDLs (very low-density lipoproteins) and LDLs (low-density lipoproteins), and high levels of HDLs (high-density lipoproteins). It is important to keep LDL cholesterol, which is an independent risk factor, below 130 mg/dl and your HDL above 35 mg/dl.

There is evidence that polyunsaturated fats (safflower, sunflower, corn, soybean and cotton seed oils) help reduce overall cholesterol without lowering your HDLs. So do monounsaturated fats like oil from olives, peanuts and avocados.

**If you're still eating a lot of** eggs, red meat, ice cream, cream, whole milk, and butter, you should be able to get a noticeable lowering by switching to skim milk, low-fat dairy products, margerine and fish, and cutting back sharply on eggs and meat.

Adding foods like oat bran, corn bran, rice bran, beans and rice could help as well.

**Regular exercise is important.** It helps increase your HDLs; a reduced HDL cholesterol level is a major risk factor.

**Keeping your weight under control,** sticking to low fat, high fiber diet and keeping blood lipids in a healthy balance is a lifelong effort. It is never too early to start.

Start now. This book will help you lead a long and healthy life.

## LOWERING YOUR BLOOD LIPID LEVELS

The key formula for lowering your serum cholesterol is, as we said, diet and exercise. If you genuinely wish to lower your serum cholesterol, and therefore lower your risk for premature heart attack, you will need to make lifestyle changes. These changes should be made in a dedicated fashion. They should be made gradually, but they must be made *permanently*.

The hard fact is that our national dietary habits are very poor as reflected in the fact that our total caloric intake is overloaded with saturated fat, cholesterol, and simple sugars. When you have an overabundance of ethanol and simple sugars in your diet you are going to elevate your triglycerides. If you have an overabundance of saturated fats in your diet you will elevate your total cholesterol, and to a lesser extent your triglycerides. As a wealthy nation, we do not pay close attention to good nutritional habits. Perhaps our comfort has lulled us into thinking that fast foods, red meat, fried foods, and processed foods represent technological advances. They don't. Excessive consumption of these food products represents ignorance about good health, laziness, and a general unwillingness to learn about good nutritional habits. In far too many instances we are more concerned about ease than we are about the quality of nutrition that will foster long life and good health. Too often we equate the most comfortable lifestyle with the most convenient, sacrificing health and vigor.

## WATCHING YOUR PROSPERITY CUES

In our society the major food products associated with prosperity are often the worst in terms of nutritional qualities. Our fancy menus dwell upon cream sauces, rich cheeses, thick steaks, lobster, shrimp. Although all of these foods are associated with prosperity and cost an inordinate amount when purchased for home preparation or in restaurants, often they are of mediocre to poor quality as nutritional supplements. For example, the primary value of red meat is the protein; the other constituents—besides vitamins and iron, when they are present—are not beneficial, and some are actually harmful.

Examine your prosperity cues. What are some of the foods that make you feel "successful"? Do they promote good health? What cues you to the success of others? Are you impressed when you are served prime rib roast of beef or filet mignon? After you have examined your general attitude toward the things that define prosperity, look very closely at the particular foods you associate with prosperity in the home and on restaurant menus. Analyze your use of fast and processed foods. Look at your reasons for using these items and the frequency of use. Do you use them for convenience? Or taste? Compare your list to what you are beginning to hear about high-quality nutrition. Begin now to learn how to equate prosperity with good nutritional products and with good health.

### *Change is Difficult*

The difficulty of changing old habits is enormous, but when it comes to reducing atherosclerotic plaque and the deadly clogging of your arteries, the imperative is urgent. Essential to lifestyle adjustments is the ability to maintain weight loss and the ability to recognize and change poor habits. The first step in this direction is to consult a cardiologist about changing your diet. Your effort will require a disciplined approach involving the eating of regular meals and planned snacks.

The prevalence of hyperlipidemia (elevated serum lipid levels) among Americans and its direct link to dietary excesses make diet modification the most rational approach to its control. Reject the attitude that changing your dietary habits is doomed to failure. Many individuals have very successfully used dietary modification to lower serum lipid levels and to achieve the loss of unwanted fat.

After your physician has given you an overview of the best therapeutic plan for your case—the role of diet, exercise, and perhaps drugs—ask him or her to assist you in reviewing your daily routine to assess your lifestyle for areas that might interfere with adherence to the plan. Ask for advice on how to modify these areas; ask your doctor to share with you how other patients have managed similar situations, and for suggestions on breaking habits that might interfere with adherence.

When you meet with your dietitian, nurses, or other health professionals, discuss your blood lipid profile and risk factors with each of them, soliciting tips on areas to be sensitive to as you try to adhere to the program. These highly skilled professionals can help you accomplish your goals. You will be surprised at the amount of helpful information you will get from them. Friends, family, and coworkers are also a rich reservoir of experiences and ideas you can tap. Avoid people who attempt to show you why it can't be done or recite ex-

Fig. 1 U.S. Prevalence of High Blood Cholesterol* by Age, Race, and Sex (Percent of Each Population)

| | Men | | Women | |
|---|---|---|---|---|
| Age, y | White | Black | White | Black |
| 20–74 | 25.0 | 23.9 | 29.2 | 23.7 |
| 20–24 | 6.1 | 2.9 | 6.5 | 7.0 |
| 25–34 | 15.0 | 19.3 | 12.4 | 8.7 |
| 35–44 | 27.9 | 24.5 | 21.1 | 16.9 |
| 45–54 | 36.5 | 40.3 | 40.6 | 40.7 |
| 55–64 | 37.3 | 35.3 | 53.7 | 46.5 |
| 65–74 | 32.4 | 27.2 | 52.1 | 48.4 |

*Serum concentration of cholesterol ≥240 mg/dl.

amples of failure. They are negative thinkers. Seek out those who are supportive of your effort and cite success stories.

It is enormously helpful at the outset to identify ways to adjust your daily routine to enhance your ability to stick to the plan. Solicit your physician's assistance in designing a self-monitoring program and ways of keeping daily records. Bring your records to each of your follow-up appointments. Review them with your doctor and listen carefully to his or her assessment of your progress. Good records will better allow your physician to offer modification tips and provide helpful support for your positive efforts. Certainly there will be times when you will do better than others. When you find yourself slipping, return immediately to the program. You must be persistent. Perseverance is a powerfully rewarding virtue.

Unfortunately there is very little societal support for prudent dietary modification. It is extremely important, therefore, to involve others in your plans. Your chances for long-term adherence and success are greatly enhanced when you openly share your plans with spouse, children, friends, and other close associates while also eliciting their support. The lack of social support can be devastating. With the proper support from your significant others, you can become a positive statistic and shining example for others.

### *Reading Labels Is a Must*

Most of us do not like to read food container labels. Therefore we are eating without knowing exactly what we are ingesting. In a real sense "we are what we eat"—and Americans eat poorly.

In Chapter 1 we discussed the importance of risk factors in diagnosing and treating high blood lipids. No sound treatment plan can be devised without first considering the risk factors involved. You saw that there are risk factors that are under your control and others that are not. For example, women are more prone to heart attack after menopause; as we age, we all become more susceptible to stroke or heart attack. (Health food advocates would argue that this age susceptibility is a direct result of the accumulation of lifelong poor dietary habits.) Perhaps the most outstanding unalterable risk factor for premature heart attack is heredity.

You are at greater risk for early cardiovascular disease if you have a positive family history of premature coronary artery disease in a first-degree relative (sibling or parent). Premature occurrence is considered to be 55 years or less.

Americans like to eat out of jars and cans; and since we do not like to read labels, we are constantly bombarded with saturated fat from palm oil and coconut oil. These oils do not easily become rancid and are used as a ubiquitous sort of preservative in all types of processed foods to extend their

Fig. 2 Risk Status Based on Presence of CHD Risk Factors Other Than LDL-Cholesterol

The patient is considered to have a high-risk status if he or she has one of the following:

- Definite CHD: the characteristic clinical picture and objective laboratory findings of either:
  - Definite prior myocardial infarction, or
  - Definite myocardial ischemia, such as angina pectoris
- Two other CHD risk factors:
  - Male sex*
  - Family history of premature CHD (definite myocardial infarction or sudden death before 55 years of age in a parent or sibling)
  - Cigarette smoking (currently smokes more than ten cigarettes per day)
  - Hypertension
  - Low HDL-cholesterol concentration (below 35 mg/dl confirmed by repeated measurement)
  - Diabetes mellitus
  - History of definite cerebrovascular or occlusive peripheral vascular disease
  - Severe obesity (≥39% overweight)

*Male sex is considered a risk factor in this scheme because the rates of CHD are three to four times higher in men than in women in the middle decades of life and roughly two times higher in the elderly. Hence, a man with one other CHD risk factor is considered to have a high-risk status, whereas a woman is not so considered unless she has two other CHD risk factors.

shelf life. If you happen to have a genetic predisposition to metabolizing cholesterol and saturated fat improperly, then you wind up with even small indiscretions—eating eggs several times per week, eating palm oil in a variety of canned and processed foods, eating fried foods—pushing your blood fat up. Minor dietary indiscretions turn into major consequences: high cholesterol and premature heart attack.

Do not carry out so important an activity as food shopping when you are rushed. Allot time to read the labels of products you are unfamiliar with. If you have not already made a habit of reading labels, you are probably unfamiliar with all of the products you are currently using. If you find the small print on labels difficult to read, purchase a small magnifying glass that will fit easily into your bag or pocket and begin to read those labels to make sure that your intake is in compliance with your cholesterol-lowering program. Many labels now indicate caloric values and a growing number are also indicating the amount of cholesterol in a product.

Start with the shelves in your own pantry. First read the nutritional information to determine if it is in line with your needs. Then go on to the very important listing of ingredients. The contents are listed in rank order by volume on food labels. Remember, if egg yolk is listed first then you are getting more egg yolk than any other ingredient. If you are looking for fiber and it is the fourth item on the ingredient list, the product is a poor choice since there are three other ingredients with greater volume than fiber.

You will want to be especially aware of a food's fat content and its position in the list of ingredients. Avoid hydrogenated vegetable oils: the hydrogenation process turns them into saturated fats, which are easily converted into cholesterol once inside your body.

## SERUM CHOLESTEROL LEVELS AND CANCER

Women with high levels of blood lipids suffer a greater incidence of breast cancer, although research has not yet indicated just why this is so.

Since the body's way of making fat soluble in blood is by attaching it to proteins and also by using bowel salts and bowel acids to aid in the solubility of its digestion, and since cholesterol and saturated fat are sticky substances, high concentrations of fat in the colon may cause the bowel acids to remain in contact with the delicate lining of the intestinal wall too long.

If your diet contains too much processed food and not enough natural fiber, there tends to be a prolonged transit time through the colon. This sluggish evacuation can result in poor health. Natural fiber and natural bulk help push waste material along, decreasing the transit time.

### Choose a High-Fiber Diet

The cells of plants, fruits, vegetables, seeds, nuts, beans, and whole grains all contain fiber. There are two classes of fiber, soluble and insoluble. Nature has amply endowed a range of food products with the matter we call insoluble fiber. Among the well-known foods that contain insoluble fiber are such products as whole wheat bran, vegetables, fruits, and whole grains. The cellulose and lignin (insoluble fibers) found in these sources prevent constipation and, according to a growing number of expert opinions, also help to prevent cancer of the colon. It is to our benefit to consume sufficient amounts of insoluble fiber. The fiber in processed and overcooked food is either damaged or destroyed, negating its potential benefit to the human body. Since insoluble fibers are not absorbed by the body, they are considered nonnutritive. Water-soluble fibers, on the other hand, are quite nutritious.

The USDA recommended requirements for dietary fiber on a daily basis range from 10 to 20 grams. Most Americans take in only 1 to 2 grams per day. So across the board in this society, we don't take in enough dietary fiber. This is true even of healthy people who don't have elevated blood lipid levels.

When eaten lightly steamed or raw, there are many green vegetables—including spinach, string beans, cabbage, celery, broccoli, collards, and greens of any sort—that will provide beneficial dietary fiber, as will the skins of fruits. Whole grain products are also excellent sources of insoluble fiber. They should be sought over processed flour products at all times. Choose whole grain cereals such as granola (since commercial granola may contain added saturated fat in the form of coconut oil, it is best to make your own) that do not have salt, sugar, or fat added. Shredded wheat is currently a popular source of dietary fiber because the USDA rates it very low in simple sugars, salt, and fat content.

Oats, dried beans, apples, oranges, and barley are abundantly supplied with fiber that will dissolve in water. This soluble fiber has received widespread media coverage and has been linked to lower cholesterol levels. The *Journal of the American Dietetic Association* reports the findings of a twelve-week study conducted at the Northwestern University Medical School in Chicago indicating that inclusion of sufficient amounts of oat fiber in the diet does indeed reduce cholesterol levels.

Oat bran seems to be the current preferred dietary fiber. It apparently has been very effective in lowering serum cholesterol. Nevertheless, oat bran's superiority has not been proven in a well-designed, double placebo study. It appears that if oat bran is to be of any help to your blood lipid–lowering program it must be taken daily in substantial volume.

A high-fiber diet is associated with the prevention of certain malignancies; it is also an independent factor in lowering serum cholesterol along with aerobic exercise, the restriction of saturated fat intake, and the cessation of cigarette smoking. The diet makes the most sense when consumed in an organic framework, however. Rather than taking products with artificial fiber, you should make every effort to get the fiber in its natural, organic state. In this way you begin to guarantee that the body handles it as naturally and as predictably as possible. The reliance on artificial fiber products may not serve your health over the long run.

Acceptance of artificial products for our bodies reflects our belief that technology is better than nature, and certainly that technology can equal nature. The use of artificial fiber in your diet may prove to be harmful. Another area where we seem to believe that technology is better than nature is in the field of artificial sweeteners. Their "superiority" resides in their ability to withstand extremes of hot and cold and a guaranteed prolonged shelf life. Their nutritional benefit is quite debatable and long-term studies may indeed prove that they have a deleterious potential. High doses of saccharin have, in fact, been shown to produce tumors. Granted, the amounts consumed by the subjects in laboratory tests were enormous. You might argue that it would take years, or perhaps more than a lifetime, to consume those amounts in your daily diet. Nevertheless, it is never wise to endure prolonged exposure to manufactured chemicals.

When it comes to your good health, it will pay to avoid artificial flavorings, colorings, and drugs designed specifically for therapeutic management. Simple sugars contain no fiber, and some experts believe they elevate triglyceride levels. Branch chain sugars (complex carbohydrates), natural sugars such as fructose, and nature's pure honey are much wiser choices as sweetening agents. The technical name for branch chain sugars is pectin. These glucose sources have a complex structure that does not permit rapid decomposition to carbon monoxide and water. Since their chemical structure is so complicated, they break down into compounds other than simple glucose. The branch chain sugars then accumulate in the liver as glycogen, which is released as it is needed when the liver senses the body's rising metabolic demand for glucose, thus maintaining stable blood sugar levels.

Although branch chain sugars are somewhat low in nutritional value, these sweeteners are stored in the liver as carbohydrates and are easier for it to handle. They are better than accumulations of simple sugars, which result in an overabundance of fatty products and wide swings in your serum insulin levels. Therefore, complex carbohydrates are the preferred source for the consumption of sugar. When simple sugars are used, avoid the varieties that are highly processed. Use natural brown sugar, molasses, and pure honey. Many people use raisins, bananas, apples, dates, figs, and other fruit as natural sweeteners.

While early and tentative research seems to indicate that the water-soluble type of fiber found in products such as oat bran, when taken in large enough amounts for a long enough period of time, serves to reduce serum cholesterol levels, we see also that insoluble fiber found in products such as wheat bran assists in the work of the colon and may decrease the risk of untimely malignancies. It is important to keep in mind that the fundamental principle of nature is balance. You will want to acquire eating habits that allow for the ingestion of balanced proportions of both soluble and insoluble fiber. Eating a wide variety of fresh, whole, nonprocessed foods increases your chance of a balanced diet. This intelligent pursuit of good nutrition ultimately increases your chances of getting all of the nutrients required for good health.

### *High-Dosage Alternatives to Proper Diet*

Most experts agree that balance and moderation are probably the best approaches to good health. We have been told since we were children that our diets should be "balanced"—red meat and dairy products were necessary to good nutrition. Now we hear that what we believed to be balanced might be deadly. One of the results of this new awareness is that we now take megadoses of vitamins, artificial fiber, the omega fatty fish acids, and many more products. Again we rush to technology rather than to the slow process of prudent dietary knowledge and control.

Vitamin supplements in megadoses and omega 3 fatty acids (fish oils) when prepared pharmacologically—by artificial means—are of little benefit and may actually pose the risk of predisposition to hemorrhaging.

High doses of vitamin A, for instance, can result in damage to several vital organs. Despite the so-called technological advances by which you can replace organic nutrients with artificial, pharmacological substitutes, it is important to understand that these substitutes are not processed by the intestines and by other necessary organs in the same way as the natural food product is.

Too many people think that they can eat processed food and then get their omega fish oils in a capsule. They mistakenly believe that at a relatively young age it is necessary to take B-vitamin supplements, excessive dosages of vitamin C, zinc, and other vitamin supplements every day. Many people do this because they know they are not getting proper nutrition from their current dietary habits. This is a very foolish way to live. Without a doubt the best way to get the vitamins, minerals, protein, and other nutrients that your body needs to sustain good health is to eat a wide variety of fresh whole foods.

The route of artificial supplementation should be saved for those circumstances where it is known that the body cannot produce the natural vitamins and organic compounds that are necessary or when some intestinal disease results in malabsorption so that the individual is not able to take in the necessary nutrients in an organic state. It is only in cases such as these that artificial means such as $B_{12}$ injections and dietary iron supplementation are called for. It is much better for an individual without absorption problems to get his or her vitamins and minerals in an organic form. This is the way the body—the liver, the intestines, and other organs—recognizes these essential nutrients.

## *Raw Vegetables: The Highest Source of Nutrition*

There is no higher form of nourishment available than raw vegetables and fruits. When fruits, vegetables, and nuts are taken in a raw, uncooked form their enzymes, minerals, vitamins, and fiber remain intact. If you eat a wide variety you are likely to get the eight amino acids required to provide your body with the fuel needed to manufacture a whole protein. The low-fat, high-fiber menus presented in Chapter 4 include an abundance of vegetable and fruit salads. Any vegetable that you like cooked can be used raw, and will add delight and zest to a salad.

Don't be timid in the preparation of your salads; experiment and find variety. It's a good idea to consume a large bowl of vegetable salad prior to your lunch and dinner meal. The sprouts from seeds, beans, grains, and nuts add flavor and nutrition to your raw vegetables. Use them liberally. Among the most nourishing and popular are alfalfa sprouts, mung beans, aduki beans, lentils, soybeans, barley, radishes, and sunflower seeds.

When vegetables are to be cooked, they are best if lightly steamed and eaten while still crunchy. This preserves their life-giving nutrients and the quality of the fiber. If you wish to sauté your vegetables occasionally, use olive oil instead of butter, and sauté them over a low heat for no more than 2 or 3 minutes. Garnish with your favorite seasoning and enjoy the natural juices that are still locked in.

## *GOOD MEDICINE AND MANAGING WHOLISTICALLY*

The Report of the National Cholesterol Education Program Expert Panel on Detection, Evaluation, and Treatment of High Blood Cholesterol in Adults repeatedly emphasizes that dietary therapy is the primary cholesterol-lowering treatment, and should be the first line of attack. The panel cautions against the early institution of drug therapy except in the most extreme cases. The goal of dietary therapy is to lower LDL cholesterol levels to below 160 mg/dl, or 130 mg/dl when there is the presence of definite coronary heart disease or two or more risk factors.

The goal of your dietary modifying program should be twofold. You must first be concerned with developing a style of eating that provides adequate to superior nutrition while reducing your cholesterol levels. If you are overweight you should also be concerned with reducing your caloric intake so that you can gradually and permanently lose your excess body fat.

With the exception of genetic predisposition, elevated blood lipids are a result of excessive consumption of the wrong kinds of food. The cure really rests on our ability and commitment as a society and as individuals to develop eating habits that modify excessive, improper consumption. Dietary therapy is the logical approach to a problem we each have so much control over.

Old habits are hard to break. Perhaps you are concerned about adjusting a new diet to your busy schedule, to your spouse or children, or to your inherently good taste that naturally leads you to favor the choicest gourmet foods. We are not advocating abrupt change, but dedicated, gradual, *permanent* change. Just keep in mind that to modify your diet so that it is a better one—and so that you can reap the results of an overall better quality of life—you do not have to give up good taste. The goal is to eat food that is good *for* you as well as good *to* you. As you restrict your fat and caloric intake, you will gradually learn ways (appropriate recipes, menus, and restaurants that cater to good health and good taste) to satisfy your palate as well as lead you to better nutrition. Keep in mind that there are over 2,000 varieties of fruits and vegetables regularly harvested on this planet! Talk to friends, relatives, business associates, and others you know who are in the process of modifying their diets or have already done so successfully. You will find that you can develop a coterie of people who offer endless suggestions on ways to accomplish your goals. You will find too that increasing numbers of recipes in magazines and newspapers indicate the amounts of calories and fatty acids, making the job of nutritional management easier.

An excellent source of healthy fatty acids is found in fish, which generally supplies polyunsaturated fat and minimal amounts of dietary cholesterol (shellfish such as lobster, crab, and shrimp, however, should be eaten only in moderate amounts; although they do contain a substantial amount of cholesterol, they are relatively low in saturated fat when compared to red meat and organ meats).

Be imaginative as you develop better dietary habits, habits that may at best prolong your life and will at least reduce the risk of premature heart attack. Draw upon all of the resources in your community to support better eating. Visit your local Weight Watchers group and obtain information on dietary modification procedures as well as new food ideas (but avoid their processed food products). Visit your local health food store and look for alternatives suitable to your taste; you might be surprised at how many things you find there that you like. Talk with the people who work there about your goals. Usually these people have an abundance of information on good eating habits. Discuss your findings with your physician and your dietitian.

Set goals and rewards for accomplishing them. Do *not* make food a reward item, however. A trip to the theater, a day to do nothing, a new record album, a massage or facial, a new hairstyle—all of these make appropriate rewards.

If you are like most of us, there will probably be times when you just won't make your goals. Analyze carefully the obstacles to your success. Meet with your physician for consultation on developing successful strategies to achieve your goals. If your total cholesterol is over 200, you may need the services of a nutritional counselor to help you implement your new strategies. Try again with a renewed commitment. It will take time to effect the modification of lifelong habits. As we've said before, your conversion to better dietary habits should be gradual and permanent.

## THE DIETARY PROGRAM

The Step-One and Step-Two diets recommended by the Expert Panel on Detection, Evaluation, and Treatment of High Blood Cholesterol in Adults are designed to progressively lower the amounts of cholesterol and saturated fatty acids you eat. Once in your body saturated fat is easily converted into cholesterol. By eliminating excess caloric intake you can also promote weight loss.

The Step-One Diet—in accordance with recommendations from the American Heart Association, the National Institutes of Health, and the U.S. Surgeon General—keeps the intake of total fat to less than 30 percent of your total calories, saturated fatty acids to less than 10 percent of your total caloric intake, and your total cholesterol intake to less than 300 mg/dl per day. Depending on the severity of your blood lipid elevation and your risk factors, your physician and/or nutritionist should monitor your progress six weeks after beginning the diet, again at three months, and at the end of six months. This book offers a 30-day program, during which time your cholesterol levels should *begin* to decrease. However, long-term results are the fruit of long-term adherence to a sound cholesterol-lowering program.

If after six months of strict adherence to your dietary plan you have no appreciable drop in your cholesterol levels, you will probably be advised to proceed to the Step-Two Diet. It is strongly recommended that when you are working on the more restrictive Step-Two Diet a registered nutritional counselor or dietitian be involved. Ask your physician to refer you to such a person. The Step-Two Diet reduces saturated fats and cholesterol to minimal levels. It allows less than 30 percent of total calories to come from fatty acids, with saturated fats representing less than 7 percent of your total caloric intake. Polyunsaturated fatty acids can represent up to 10 percent of your total caloric intake and monounsaturated fatty acids can represent 10 to 15 percent of your total calories. Consult the chart below for a detailed analysis of each diet.

Remember, saturated fatty acids and cholesterol are not essential nutrients and are not, therefore, requirements for a healthy human diet. They come into our diets as a result of acquired taste. Your magnificent body machine can produce an abundance of these lipids naturally when you are in good health.

Since the goal of the diet is to reduce "major and obvious" sources of fatty acid and cholesterol, it will be helpful if you begin to keep a very detailed food record. This record will help you, your doctor, and/or your registered dietitian plan a program that best suits your needs. Purchase a small notebook, one that you can keep handy at all times. For seven days prior to your first meeting with the registered dietitian, record every item you consume in a day from the time you get up to bedtime. If you have a habit of raiding the refrigerator at 3:00 A.M., record all that you eat. Be as exact as you can in describing the size and amount of the portions. At the

Fig. 3 Dietary Therapy of High Blood Cholesterol Level

| Nutrient | Recommended Intake | |
|---|---|---|
| | Step-One Diet | Step-Two Diet |
| Total Fat | Less than 30% of total calories | Less than 30% of total calories |
| Saturated fatty acids | Less than 10% of total calories | Less than 7% of total calories |
| Polyunsaturated fatty acids | Up to 10% of total calories | Up to10% of total calories |
| Monounsaturated fatty acids | 10% to 15% of total calories | 10% to 15% of total calories |
| Carbohydrates | 50% to 60% of total calories | 50% to 60% of total calories |
| Protein | 10% to 20% of total calories | 10% to 20% of total calories |
| Cholesterol | Less than 300 mg/dl | Less than 200 mg/dl |
| Total calories | To achieve and maintain desirable weight | To achieve and maintain desirable weight |

same time write down your motivation for the eating. Are you eating because you are hungry or because it is your usual mealtime? Are you eating because you are frustrated? Excited? Bored? Depressed? Worried? To be social? This information will be of enormous help to you as you attempt to modify your eating habits as well as aiding your doctor and your dietitian in developing appropriate strategies for achieving your goals.

### *Monitoring Adherence and Results*

Obviously, the key to the success of any program of behavior modification is adherence to the terms of the plan. If you have accomplished your goals at any one of the checkpoints, you then enter a long-term monitoring program. During the first year your adherence and blood levels should be assessed quarterly; thereafter, twice yearly. These regular consultations with your physician and registered dietitian will be of enormous benefit in assisting you in maintaining your long-term commitment. It is not at all unusual to begin to slip back into old habits after meeting your goals. How many pounds have you lost and then regained? Similarly, you will need to keep your cholesterol levels down permanently. Regular consultations will keep you alert to your patterns and to back-sliding.

If you have minimal risk factors, have previously obtained a total cholesterol count and a fasting lipid profile, it is not necessary to do a third fasting to determine the adequacy or results of dietary and exercise modifications; according to the National Institutes of Health report on serum cholesterol, this applies to people who fall in the low-risk group (mild or borderline elevations of serum cholesterol). The third and all succeeding tests to monitor your progress if you fall in the above categories can be nonfasting tests that focus on total cholesterol counts and the levels of the deadly LDL cholesterol.

If your total LDLs are over 160 mg/dl, and you have two risk factors, it is prudent to monitor your blood lipid levels using a 12- to 14-hour fasting cholesterol sample. Earlier you saw that among the eleven risk factors for coronary heart disease are male sex, an elevated cholesterol total, positive family history of premature coronary heart disease, severe obesity (above 30 percent of your ideal body weight), cigarette smoking, and diabetes. If you possess two or more of the eleven previously listed risks, then the numbers for aggressive management of your cholesterol profile need to be scaled downward. It then makes sense to use a total cholesterol count of 200 and an LDL of 130 mg/dl. A total cholesterol count of 240 mg/dl corresponds roughly to an LDL total of 160 mg/dl, while a serum cholesterol total of 200 corresponds roughly to 130 mg/dl.

Since your cholesterol-lowering program will be based on your blood lipid levels, it is critical to know that the laboratory you are using has a standard deviation on a fasting cholesterol test of no more than 10 percent. Although it will not give you an absolute level from test to test or from specimen to specimen, when the standard deviation is held to 10 percent you can be comfortable in knowing that you have a reasonable picture of what your cholesterol trend is and that your lowering program is accurate.

The degree of exactitude required in your lab testing if you possess multiple risk factors and a dramatically elevated serum cholesterol and LDL cholesterol count becomes more important. Keep in mind that the absolute number is not necessarily the important issue, what is important is the degree of relative coronary risk based upon your LDL and your risk factors. Therefore, if you have two or more risk factors, if your total cholesterol is above 240 mg/dl, and if your LDL cholesterol is above 160 mg/dl, it is prudent to obtain fasting levels with a standard deviation of less than 10 percent for your monitoring the assessment of program accuracy.

If your cholesterol goals are not met three months into the Step-One Diet, you should continue it for an additional three months, unless your doctor feels that you are at too great a risk. If at the end of six months on the Step-One Diet you still have not achieved your goals, proceed to the Step-Two program, a more restrictive regimen. Again, your adherence and levels should be assessed within four to six weeks, after three months,, and finally at the end of six months. If at the end of this six-month period on the Step-Two Diet your levels have not fallen sufficiently to bring you into safe ranges, your doctor may need to consider more aggressive management by drug therapy. In all but the most extreme cases, the Expert Panel recommends at least a year of proven dietary adherence before introducing drug therapy.

However, drug therapy should be considered at the end of six months if the LDL is markedly elevated. If the LDL count is greater than or equal to 190 mg/dl in a male patient at the end of six months of strict adherence to a sequential Step-One and Step-Two diet, that patient should be started on appropriate drug therapy.

What an expert will decide to do to manage a case of borderline hypercholesterolemia depends predominantly upon the individual's age and sex. For example, if a male patient between the ages of 20 and 29 has a total cholesterol between 200 and 220 mg/dl, many experts would place that patient on the Step-One Diet for three to six months for observation, with a repeat testing of the total cholesterol at the end of that six-month period. There are other experts who would additionally advocate that a young patient in this category have a lipid profile performed to measure the total LDL cholesterol.

On the other hand, if a patient is between the ages of 30 and 39 and has a total cholesterol of 220 to 240 without the presence of any other risk factors, many experts would place this individual on the Step-One Diet, measuring the patient's LDL at the initiation of treatment.

If an elderly female patient has an LDL cholesterol of greater than 160 mg/dl but less than 190, one would not consider the initiation of drug treatment but would use consistent dietary management with the Step-One Diet for as long as possible. In elderly women it is very important that adequate protein and caloric content be maintained, and only the most severe cases of LDL elevation should be considered for drug therapy and the Step-Two Diet.

Male patients without any other risk factors who have a borderline high total cholesterol of between 200 and 240 should have a lipid profile drawn and be managed with aggressive dietary therapy.

If poor adherence to the diet is the only reason your lipid levels have not fallen sufficiently, before entering drug therapy you should enroll in a behavioral modification program. You should make every effort to control your blood fats without medication. Anyway, drug therapy does not free you of your responsibility to adhere to the diet, since drug therapy is always used in conjunction with the diet.

### When to Introduce Drugs: The Risk

> *The decision for drug therapy is a serious one. All of the drugs on today's market to lower serum cholesterol have side effects. There is not one drug that is more free of side effects than another. The decision for drug therapy should be made knowing that the result is clearly beneficial to the patient and vastly outweighs the risk.*
>
> —Dr. Alan Beckles

Louis, a 64-year-old automobile salesman, was totally asymptomatic when he visited his doctor, although he had a markedly positive family history of premature coronary disease. For five years he had known that he had a moderate to marked elevation in his serum cholesterol total. However, Louis had never been placed on a supervised low-fat, low-cholesterol diet.

Because his treadmill exercise test was abnormal, the doctor gave him a thallium imaging exercise test—this treadmill test has a greater degree of sensitivity—which was also abnormal. Next he gave Louis a coronary angiography to determine the location and the extent of coronary atherosclerosis; it demonstrated a totally occluded coronary artery. Fortunately, Louis had developed a good collateral flow (the formation of tiny vessels that shunt the blood around the blocked area), which prevented scarring of his heart muscle.

Despite strict adherence to the Step-One Diet for three months, Louis's cholesterol value remains at 250 mg/dl. The addition of cholestyramine or niacin will be considered on his next visit if there is not a substantial drop in his serum cholesterol level. It is not unusual in cases of positive family history to find that diet, even with strict adherence, will not sufficiently lower the patient's totals, making drug therapy a necessity.

Nevertheless, prudence is the watchword when drug therapy is applied. With a menopausal woman, the benefits of aggressively lowering her cholesterol from a markedly elevated level with drug therapy might not really prolong health or prevent coronary disease in a way that makes it worth the aggressive management of drug therapy. In such a patient dietary manipulation should be pushed to its utmost and drug therapy reserved to the most benign agent available after holding back as long as possible.

The tolerance for initiation of drug therapy in individual patients should be based upon age and risk factors. A young man would probably be considered for drug therapy if after six months to a year on aggressive dietary management and modification of risk factors he still demonstrates a total cholesterol above 240 and an LDL above 160. However, if that young man has another risk factor in addition to his sex, every effort should be made to achieve a 200 mg/dl total cholesterol count and LDL values of 130 mg/dl. If this cannot be achieved nonpharmacologically, then drug therapy should be instituted.

The aggressiveness with which an elevated cholesterol is pursued and rectified to a significant degree depends on the judgments of the physician and nutritionist. Even with the classic middle-aged male who has a high cholesterol level and one other risk factor, or the relatively young patient who may have multiple risk factors such as a significant genetic risk for coronary heart disease and high blood pressure, at least six months of dietary therapy should always be tried first.

The first three months for patients in this category are restricted to the Step-One Diet. Since people in this category are at greater risk, if after three months on the Step-One Diet the patient does not show sufficient falls in blood lipid levels, the Step-Two Diet is instituted. Only after ascertaining that the patient has adhered strictly to the daily meal plan should drug therapy be considered. And even in that instance niacin may well be the drug of first choice. Most patients have a mixed elevation of the lipids cholesterol and triglycerides; for these people, niacin, which is the most organic of the drugs available, is the drug of first choice.

The duration of treatment on either the Step-One or Step-Two Diet before intervention with pharmacological agents depends upon the presence of risk factors and the patient's age.

Drug therapy may be initiated in adult patients who despite prolonged strict adherence to dietary therapy still have LDL cholesterol levels of: 1) 190+ mg/dl (if they do not have definite coronary heart disease or two other risk factors, one of which can be male sex; an individual with LDL cholesterol levels of this magnitude is at very high risk of developing CHD); 2) 160+ mg/dl (if they have definite CHD or two other risk factors).

Medical discretion is required in using these guidelines. While men with LDL cholesterol values between 160 and 190 mg/dl who have any other risk factor are primary candidates for drug therapy, it might be far less desirable in older women. Since the absolute risk of CHD is lower in women than in men, the approach to drug therapy for females is usually conservative.

If maximum dietary modification were practiced by society at large we would see a significant decrease in the percentage of both men and women being considered for drug therapy. The first attack on elevated blood lipids should be nonpharmacological, with emphasis placed on diet, weight control, exercise, cessation of cigarette smoking, elimination of or effective coping with stress, and other lifestyle modifications.

Low-density lipoprotein cholesterol is the best barometer for making decisions to initiate drug therapy and for the monitoring of the response to the therapy. Without a doubt the decision to use drugs is always a guarded one, since the commitment may be for years or for the duration of the individual's life.

The goals of drug therapy are the same as those of dietary therapy: to lower LDLs to 160 mg/dl for those without diagnosed coronary heart disease or two other risk factors, one of which can be male sex; to lower LDLs to 130 mg/dl in those with definite CHD or two other risk factors. Although more research is required to establish exact LDL levels to promote regression of atherosclerotic plaque, many experts believe that LDL levels of 100 mg/dl and below is an ideal goal.

At present the major drugs in use are the bile acid sequestrants (cholestyramine and colestipol); nicotinic acid (niacin); and HMG-CoA-Reductase inhibitors (Lovastatin, Gemfibrozil, and Probucol). See the chart on page 59.

Fig. 4 Calculated Levels of Serum Low-Density Lipoprotein (LDL) Cholesterol* for Persons† 20 to 74 Years of Age Fasting 12 Hours or More, by Sex and Age: Means and Selected Percentiles, United States, 1976–1980

| Sex, Age, y | No. of Persons Examined | Estimated Population In Thousands | Mean | SD | Selected Percentiles 5th | 10th | 15th | 25th | 50th | 75th | 85th | 90th | 95th |
|---|---|---|---|---|---|---|---|---|---|---|---|---|---|
| Men | | | | | | | | | | | | | |
| 20–74 | 1037 | 21262 | 140 | 39 | 80 | 92 | 100 | 113 | 136 | 164 | 181 | 194 | 208 |
| 20–24 | 72 | 1852 | 109 | 36 | ‡ | 70 | 74 | 88 | 104 | 129 | 149 | 154 | ‡ |
| 25–34 | 174 | 5186 | 128 | 33 | 76 | 87 | 94 | 108 | 128 | 148 | 161 | 171 | 189 |
| 35–44 | 130 | 3866 | 145 | 40 | 81 | 96 | 105 | 116 | 138 | 176 | 192 | 203 | 206 |
| 45–54 | 106 | 3543 | 150 | 36 | 99 | 103 | 112 | 119 | 146 | 171 | 189 | 195 | 211 |
| 55–64 | 267 | 3943 | 148 | 39 | 84 | 101 | 108 | 118 | 147 | 171 | 191 | 206 | 217 |
| 65–74 | 288 | 2872 | 149 | 40 | 87 | 105 | 109 | 120 | 144 | 174 | 188 | 199 | 217 |
| Women | | | | | | | | | | | | | |
| 20–74 | 1246 | 27102 | 141 | 43 | 81 | 91 | 98 | 110 | 136 | 164 | 186 | 199 | 220 |
| 20–24 | 105 | 3325 | 114 | 33 | 69 | 74 | 83 | 94 | 106 | 136 | 149 | 155 | 179 |
| 25–34 | 194 | 5517 | 121 | 33 | 72 | 83 | 90 | 98 | 116 | 139 | 154 | 166 | 187 |
| 35–44 | 166 | 4800 | 129 | 34 | 78 | 90 | 97 | 107 | 126 | 150 | 163 | 171 | 191 |
| 45–54 | 168 | 5155 | 157 | 45 | 94 | 104 | 116 | 125 | 156 | 184 | 200 | 213 | 226 |
| 55–64 | 282 | 4644 | 159 | 42 | 101 | 113 | 118 | 129 | 150 | 188 | 205 | 219 | 237 |
| 65–74 | 331 | 3661 | 162 | 44 | 98 | 109 | 122 | 135 | 158 | 186 | 207 | 226 | 245 |

*Serum LDL Cholesterol = Serum Total Cholesterol – HDL Cholesterol – (Triglycerides/5). Equation from Friedewald et al. Persons with a serum triglyceride value greater than 400 mg/dl were excluded. From the National Center for Health Statistics: Division of Health Examination Statistics, unpublished data from the second National Health and Nutrition Examination Survey, 1976–1980.

†Includes other races in addition to black and white.

‡Sample size insufficient to produce statistically reliable results.

**Fig. 5 Initial Classification and Recommended Follow-up Based on Total Cholesterol***

| | |
|---|---|
| Classification, mg/dl | |
| <200 | Desirable blood cholesterol |
| 200 to 239 | Borderline–high blood cholesterol |
| ≥240 | High blood cholesterol |
| Recommended follow-up | |
| Total cholesterol, <200 mg/dl | Repeat within five years |
| Total cholesterol, 200–239 mg/dl | |
| *Without* definite CHD or two other CHD risk factors (one of which can be male sex) | Dietary information and recheck annually |
| *With* definite CHD or two other CHD risk factors (one of which can be male sex) | Lipoprotein analysis; further action based on LDL cholesterol level |
| Total cholesterol ≥240 mg/dl | |

*CHD indicates coronary heart disease; LDL, low-density lipoprotein.

**Fig. 6 Classification and Treatment Decisions Based on LDL-Cholesterol***

| | | |
|---|---|---|
| Classification, mg/dl | | |
| <130 | Desirable LDL cholesterol | |
| 130 to 159 | Borderline–high-risk LDL cholesterol | |
| ≥160 | High-risk LDL cholesterol | |

| | Initiation Level, mg/dl | Minimal Goal, mg/dl |
|---|---|---|
| Dietary treatment | | |
| *Without* CHD or two other risk factors† | ≥160 | <160‡ |
| *With* CHD or two other risk factors† | ≥130 | <130§ |
| Drug treatment | | |
| *Without* CHD or two other risk factors† | ≥190 | <160 |
| *With* CHD or two other risk factors† | ≥160 | <130 |

*LDL indicates low-density lipoprotein; CHD, coronary heart disease.

†Patients have a lower initiation level and goal if they are at high risk because they already have definite CHD, or because they have any two of the following risk factors: male sex, family history of premature CHD, cigarette smoking, hypertension, low high-density lipoprotein (HDL) cholesterol, diabetes mellitus, definite cerebrovascular or peripheral vascular disease, or severe obesity.

‡Roughly equivalent to total cholesterol level of <240 mg/dl or <200 mg/dl.

§As goals for monitoring dietary treatment.

Fig. 7 Summary of the Major Drugs for Consideration*

| Drugs | Reduce CHD Risk | Long-term Safety | Maintaining Adherence | LDL Cholesterol Lowering, % | Special Precautions |
|---|---|---|---|---|---|
| Cholestyramine, colestipol | Yes | Yes | Requires considerable education | 15–30 | Can alter absorption of other drugs, can increase triglyceride levels and should not be used in patients with hypertriglyceridemia |
| Nicotinic acid | Yes | Yes | Requires considerable education | 15–30 | Test for hyperuricemia, hyperglycemia, and liver function abnormalities |
| Lovastatin† | Not proven | Not established | Relatively easy | 25–45 | Monitor for liver function abnormalities, and possible lens opacities |
| Gemfibrozil‡ | Not proven | Preliminary evidence | Relatively easy | 5–15 | May increase LDL cholesterol in hypertriglyceridemic patients; should not be used in patients with gallbladder disease |
| Probucol | Not proven | Not established | Relatively easy | 10–15 | Lowers HDL cholesterol; significance of this has not been established; prolongs QT interval |

*CHD indicates coronary heart disease; LDL, low-density lipoprotein; and HDL, high-density lipoprotein.
†Recently approved by the Food and Drug Administration for marketing.
‡Not approved by the Food and Drug Administration for routine use in lowering cholesterol. The results of the Helsinki Heart Study should be available soon to define the effect on CHD risk and long-term safety.

Fig. 8 Drugs Highly Effective in Lowering LDL Cholesterol*

| Drug | Starting Dose | Maximum Dose | Usual Time and Frequency | Side Effects | Monitoring |
|---|---|---|---|---|---|
| Cholestyramine, colestipol | 4 g twice daily, 5 g twice daily | 24 g/d, 30 g/d | Twice daily, within an hour of major meals | Dose-dependent upper and lower gastrointestinal tract | Dosing schedules of coadministered drugs |
| Nicotinic acid | 100–250 mg as single dose | 3 g/d, rarely doses up to 6 g are used | Three times a day with meals to minimize flushing | Flushing, upper gastrointestinal tract and hepatic | Uric acid, liver function, glucose |
| Lovastatin | 20 mg once daily with evening meal | 80 mg/d | Once (evening) or twice daily with meals | Gastrointestinal tract and hepatic, miscellaneous, including muscle pain | Liver function, creatine kinase, lens |

*LDL indicates low-density lipoprotein.

The class of drugs called the bile acid sequestrants reduces LDLs by encouraging their removal through the intestines by binding the acids and by stimulating LDL receptor activity. A major advantage of the sequestrants is the availability of long-term safety information. The sequestrants are particularly suitable for women considering pregnancy and for children.

Cholestyramine, popularly known by the brand name Questran, reduces LDLs by helping to get rid of bile acids that contain cholesterol by removing them from the body's cells and allowing them to flow to the intestines. This results in an increase in LDL receptor activity in the liver, which promotes removal of LDL from the bloodstream. It is a powdery substance that must be mixed with water or fruit juice. The side effects include a bad taste, constipation, nausea, bloating, and inhibition of the body's ability to absorb vitamins A, D, and K, beta-blockers, and many other drugs, and increased triglyceride levels.

Colestipol, known by the brand name Colestid, also substantially lowers LDL cholesterol totals. It increases triglycerides to a lesser degree than does cholestyramine. Its side effects include nausea, constipation, bloating, and decreased ability to absorb vitamins A, D, and K and many other drugs.

The drug of first choice in lowering LDLs is niacin (nicotinic acid). The least costly of the first-choice drugs, niacin has been used for many years to lower serum lipid elevation. Niacin is one of the B-complex vitamins, $B_3$, and should not be confused with nicotinamide or niacinamide.

Niacin is a very valuable drug in the treatment of hypercholesterolemia where there is also an elevation of serum triglycerides above 240 mg/dl. Nevertheless, niacin is not a totally benign form of treatment; it does have side effects and some individuals who take it in large doses may experience dry skin, intestinal disorders, and to a lesser degree liver dysfunction.

The unpleasant experience of severe skin flushing causes many people to reject treatment with niacin. Nicotinic acid is a highly effective drug of proven efficacy and safety, so that the effort and education required to use it are justified. Flushing can be decreased by pretreatment with simple aspirin or nonsteroidal anti-inflammatory drugs. In most people tolerance to the flushing develops within a few weeks. Sustained-release products such as Nico-Bid and Endur-Acin also serve to inhibit flushing. However, the timed-release preparations cost far more than the traditional forms of nicotinic acid.

HMG-CoA-Reductase inhibitors are a new class of drugs; the most popular, known by the brand name Lovastatin, increases the LDL receptors by interacting with the enzyme HMG-CoA-Reductase to inhibit the formation of cholesterol in the liver. This activity results in lowered LDL levels and increased HDL levels. This drug has not been in use long enough to yield long-term side effect profiles; it should therefore be used with caution. This class of drugs is not as effective when used as a single agent and so is best used in combination with another drug. The side effects include gastrointestinal tract and hepatic disturbances, including muscle pain and possible liver dysfunction.

The class of drugs called fibric acid derivatives is used mainly in cases of elevated serum triglycerides. You can see from the name of the drugs that they act similarly to natural fiber that can be obtained through dietary ingestion. Before resorting to use of these drugs, be certain that you cannot use dietary modification with high fiber intake, perhaps combined with niacin, to achieve desirable cholesterol levels.

When the response to a single drug is inadequate, it is common for cholesterol-lowering drugs to be used in combinations to achieve greater reductions and decreased side effects. Combined drug treatment involves using two agents with synergistic mechanisms of action. It is advisable to consult a lipid specialist before beginning such treatment since there is limited experience with combined drug treatment.

Rod, a 52-year-old businessman with a dramatically elevated total fasting cholesterol of 500 mg/dl, was referred to Dr. Beckles for a thallium imaging exercise study. He complained of pain in his right leg when walking. Despite his dangerously high cholesterol total, Rod had never been placed on a low-fat, low-cholesterol diet. His initial exercise treadmill stress test was aborted prematurely because he complained of leg pain. Subsequent tests revealed severe coronary artery disease. The pain in his right leg was a result of poor circulation.

Rod's condition was so severe it required a three-vessel coronary artery bypass operation, which was successful. Rod is scheduled for a bypass grafting procedure in the right leg to restore arterial flow and relieve the pain.

Dr. Beckles has placed Rod on the low-fat, low-cholesterol Step-One Diet and the synergistic combination of cholestyramine and Lovastatin. With good adherence, Rod's cholesterol is now approximately 240 mg/dl.

No doubt, had Rod implemented dietary modification much earlier in his life he might have avoided the very serious surgical procedure he underwent.

Drug therapy, like dietary therapy, will require your adherence if it is to lower your blood lipid levels successfully. After your physician has discussed with you the treatment plan, its rationale, and possible side effects, review your daily routine with him or her to identify factors in your life that could interfere with your ability to adhere to the prescribed regimen. Ask your doctor and each member of the medical team you consult for very specific suggestions and tips on adherence. It is enormously helpful at the outset to identify ways to adjust your daily activities to enhance your ability to adhere to the regimen.

Ask your physician to assist you in developing a monitoring plan and to review your records at the follow-up sessions. At this time your physician can offer helpful hints on ways to improve your ability to follow the prescribed guidelines.

It is extremely important to involve your family and friends in your regimen. These people can be enormously supportive in helping you to maintain and achieve your goals. Lack of appropriate social support can in fact be destructive when you are trying to initiate lifestyle changes that are a matter of life or death.

Determining the best approach for managing your blood lipid levels to decrease the risk of premature heart attack is a shared effort. It is partly the responsibility of a team of professionals including physicians, dietitians, nurses, and other health professionals who will participate in helping you achieve your goals. But perhaps the most challenging responsibility is yours: to make the dietary and other lifestyle changes that your program calls for.

## *THE MAINTENANCE PROGRAM*

The long-term goal of your cholesterol-lowering program is to achieve and maintain normal blood lipid levels. The cornerstones of this cholesterol-reduction program are diet, exercise, and risk modification.

The Maintenance Program, which is the core of the program for lowering your blood lipid levels, is a low-fat, high-fiber diet. It is for people who have desirable levels and wish to maintain them.

You read earlier that a desirable cholesterol is defined as anything less than 200 mg/dl on a fasting sample when the patient has been fasting for at least 12 to 14 hours. Levels between 200 and 240 (borderline high) should be treated by dietary restriction in general, but in the young male patient who may or may not have additional risk factors, drug therapy may be necessary. In the absence of other risk factors and in the absence of definite coronary heart disease, you should go on a supervised diet that limits your total cholesterol intake to no more than 300 milligrams a day; your fat intake should be limited to 3 grams or less; and the ratio of saturated fat to unsaturated fat should be less than 30 percent. Your ingestion of saturated fat must be limited because saturated fat is easily converted into cholesterol.

The unique feature of the cholesterol-lowering program is its individualized treatment. An individualized treatment based on age, risk factors, and blood values is the proper approach for lowering blood lipids. Stratifying risk according to age, risk factors, and serum levels personalizes the program presented here.

An intelligent adherence to the proper dietary habits, along with aerobic exercise and cessation of cigarette smoking, can result in a significant reduction in elevated serum cholesterol count in a large majority of people.

The menus you will find at the end of this book are to be used based on acceptable milligrams of fat content and on caloric value, depending on your individual requirements. There is an intimate relationship between body fat and serum cholesterol. You will want to watch your calories until you have lowered excess body weight to within 10 percent of your ideal weight. Exercise is critical to this program: Aerobic exercise alone can reduce your lipid levels by 10 percent.

**DESIRABLE LEVELS**
**OF BLOOD LIPIDS, CHOLESTEROL, AND TRIGLYCERIDES**

| | |
|---|---|
| Total cholesterol | 200 mg/dl and below |
| LDL cholesterol | 130 mg/dl and below |
| HDL cholesterol | 35 mg/dl and above |
| Triglycerides | 250 mg/dl and below |

If you already have desirable levels, a lifestyle that maintains low levels of serum cholesterol should be a lifelong attitude, one that ideally begins in childhood.

Perhaps your blood lipid profile reveals amounts consistent with these ranges. You will want to assure that your lipid levels are not elevated over the ensuing years by evaluating your present eating habits and making adjustments in any areas that put you at risk for potentially consuming too much saturated fat and cholesterol. You will also want to assure that you are getting enough aerobic exercise. The following indications will help you safeguard your desirable levels. These maintenance recommendations are central to the basic program for adults 20 years or older who wish to safeguard their desirable ranges.

To obtain an accurate measurement of your daily food intake, refer to *The Barbara Kraus Cholesterol Counter* and *The Barbara Kraus Calorie Counter*. Begin by increasing your fiber intake to reflect the 10 to 20 grams per day recommended by the USDA. You will also want to restrict meals that include red meat to no more than 14 percent of your total nutritional intake. This means that out of seven dinners only one should contain red meat and that should be a very lean cut with all fat trimmed away. As you trim the fat away, reducing your ingestion of saturated fatty acids, keep in mind there is still cholesterol in the cells of the lean meat. Trimming has reduced your intake of saturated fat and cholesterol, but not eliminated it.

Instead of red meat use sources of protein that are not as high in saturated fat. Fish, skinned chicken, dried peas and beans, soybean products (tofu is the most notable) are all excellent alternative sources of protein. Begin to learn more about the use of these items in your meal planning. For instance, one woman consulted a recipe book that offered 500 tasty tofu recipes and introduced to her family's delight, this fine source of protein.

Restrict your intake of dairy products, especially egg yolks. When consuming milk, yogurt, or cheese, use low-fat varieties. Avoid ice cream. You may eat sherbet occasionally, but have as many frozen fruit bars as prudent intake will allow. Eat lots of fresh fruits and vegetables every day.

Avoid snacks, allowing yourself no more than two a day. Never snack impulsively, but plan your snacks around nutritious foods: Whole wheat bagels, graham crackers, melba toast, rye crisp, oat bran muffins, granola, carrot sticks, celery, apples, oranges, bananas, unsalted nuts, frozen fruit bars, fresh-squeezed fruit or vegetable juice, and dried fruit all make wholesome snacks.

Select an assortment of your favorite fresh fruits, vegetables, nuts and seeds, and dried fruit. Chop the fresh fruit and veggies—do not mix—into bite-size pieces and put them into sandwich bags. Store the fruit and veggies in your refrigerator and the nuts and dried fruit in a cool place. Put a few in your desk drawer at work, and take along a fresh pack of fruit and vegetable bites every day. Take these handy little packets to the park or to the movies. After a while your taste buds will come to prefer your new style of snacking.

Decrease your use of highly saturated fats and oils. Butterfat, beef fat, lard, and bacon grease are all cholesterol-raising fats and should be avoided. Avoid food products containing coconut oil, palm oil, and palm kernel oil. You will want to limit the use of unsaturated vegetable oils if you are concerned about your caloric intake, since they are high in calories. Refer to *The Barbara Kraus Caloric Counter* for exact figures.

Substitute whole wheat breads, cereals, pasta, brown rice, and dried peas and beans for fatty foods. For dessert eat fruit, low-fat yogurt, sherbet, angel food cake, or Jell-O.

Food preparation is also an important consideration. The healthiest methods are steaming, baking, broiling, or grilling, which allow the fat to drip away. You may stir-fry or sauté foods occasionally.

When eating out order entrees without sauces or butter. When you are served huge portions of meat, eat only half. If you are as concerned about waste as you are about your long-term good health, then take home the excess for a later meal. But learn to eat with moderation. Avoid fast foods, processed foods, organ meats, and shellfish.

Aerobic exercise should be practiced by everyone who is orthopedically able at least three times a week for 30 minutes continuously. The goal is to push your heart rate up to approximately 70 to 75 percent of the maximum heart rate for your age. The maximum heart rate predicted for age is obtained by subtracting your age from 220. If you are 35 years old, your maximum rate is 185 beats per minute. Forms of aerobic exercise you might consider include swimming for at least 45 yards per minute for 30 minutes, riding a stationary bicycle, exercising on a track, or walking distances of at least 3 to 5 miles three to five times a week at a rate of 1 city block per minute. The aerobically fit heart takes a longer time to increase in beats per minute—thus to reach desired levels.

Analyze the risk factors presented earlier and modify any that appear in your own life. For example, if you smoke get counseling on how to quit permanently. All risk factors under your control must be modified to safeguard your desirable totals over the long run.

Remember: Low fat, high fiber, and regular aerobic exercise are *pro* life!

# 3
# Reducing Cholesterol: The Basic Dietary Plan

The Step-One Diet involves an intake of total fat less than 30 percent of total calories, saturated fat less than 10 percent of total calories, and cholesterol less than 300 mg/dl.

The Step-Two Diet is used when the response to the Step-One Diet is insufficient. While your overall intake of fat remains at 30 percent of total calories, it calls for a reduction in saturated fatty acids to less than 7 percent of total calories and in cholesterol to less than 200 mg/dl.

After you begin the Step-One Diet, your serum cholesterol should be measured and your adherence to the diet evaluated at the end of six weeks and again at the end of three months. If you have achieved your goals at either of these checkpoints, you will then enter the long-term maintenance phase in which your adherence and cholesterol totals are monitored on a quarterly basis for the first year and semiannually thereafter.

If at the end of the first three months your cholesterol levels are still high and your adherence has not been sufficient, remain on the diet and practice stricter adherence. If after three to six months of strict adherence (depending on your elevation, age, and risk factors) your lipid levels have not fallen appreciably, proceed to the Step-Two Diet. As in the Step-One phase, after six weeks your cholesterol and adherence should be monitored. If after three months on the Step-Two Diet you have two or more risk factors, an LDL total of 225 mg/dl and your levels have not fallen, drug therapy should be considered.

Jan, a 50-year-old morbidly obese woman registered a total cholesterol of 400 mg/dl. Her physical examination revealed markedly decreased peripheral arterial pulses, an indication of atherosclerosis in her lower extremities. She was immediately placed on the Step-One Diet with an 1800-calorie limitation for weight reduction. Since there is no positive family history of coronary heart disease, with strict adherence Jan should experience gradual and permanent weight loss and lowering of her cholesterol totals.

## THE FOOD YOU EAT

### Red Meat

Pork, beef, and lamb should be eaten in moderation. When they are eaten, the amount of marbling should be carefully observed and kept to a minimum, and all excess fat should be trimmed from the meat. The meat should be cooked in a manner that will allow the fat to drip away. It is very important even for people who have desirable blood lipid levels to follow these measures. We all take in too much fat. There needs to be a daily check in your mind of the last time you ate food high in saturated fat and cholesterol content. Be aware of your intake so that you can properly limit it.

### Processed Meat

Avoid bacon, hot dogs, salami, bologna, liverwurst, sausage (including Vienna sausages and pepperoni), and canned

**Fig. 9 Dietary Therapy of High Blood Cholesterol Level**

| Nutrient | Recommended Intake | |
|---|---|---|
| | Step-One Diet | Step-Two Diet |
| Total fat | Less than 30% of total calories | Less than 30% of total calories |
| Saturated fatty acids | Less than 10% of total calories | Less than 7% of total calories |
| Polyunsaturated fatty acids | Up to 10% of total calories | Up to 10% of total calories |
| Monounsaturated fatty acids | 10% to 15% of total calories | 10% to 15% of total calories |
| Carbohydrates | 50% to 60% of total calories | 50% to 60% of total calories |
| Protein | 10% to 20% of total calories | 10% to 20% of total calories |
| Cholesterol | Less than 300 mg/dl | Less than 200 mg/dl |
| Total calories | To achieve and maintain desirable weight | To achieve and maintain desirable weight |

Fig. 10 Cholesterol and Fat Content of Animal Products In Three-Ounce Portions (Cooked)

| Source | Cholesterol Content, mg/3 oz | Total Fat Content, g/3 oz |
|---|---|---|
| Red meats (lean) | | |
| Beef | 77 | 8.7 |
| Lamb | 78 | 8.8 |
| Pork | 79 | 11.1 |
| Veal | 128 | 4.7 |
| Organ meats | | |
| Liver | 270 | 4.0 |
| Pancreas (sweetbreads) | 400 | 2.8 |
| Kidney | 329 | 2.9 |
| Brains | 1746 | 10.7 |
| Heart | 164 | 4.8 |
| Poultry | | |
| Chicken (without skin) | | |
| Light | 72 | 3.8 |
| Dark | 79 | 8.2 |
| Turkey (without skin) | | |
| Light | 59 | 1.3 |
| Dark | 72 | 6.1 |
| Fish | | |
| Salmon | 74 | 9.3 |
| Tuna (light, canned in water) | 55 | 0.7 |
| Shellfish | | |
| Abalone | 90 | 0.8 |
| Clams | 57 | 1.7 |
| Crab meat | | |
| Alaskan king | 45 | 1.3 |
| Blue crab | 85 | 1.5 |
| Lobster | 61 | 0.5 |
| Oysters | 93 | 4.2 |
| Scallops | 35 | 0.8 |
| Shrimp | 166 | 0.9 |

meats. These meat products contain huge amounts of fat and are generally low in nutritional value as well.

### *Eggs*

Even if you are a person with desirable serum cholesterol levels, you should eat eggs no more than once or twice a week. Do not eat fried or scrambled eggs. Boiled and poached eggs with no addition of fat are preferable. You may eat the cholesterol-free egg whites as often as you like. Two whites are equal in calories to one whole egg.

### *Dairy Products*

Pay close attention to your consumption of all of those very fatty dairy products that our society equates with good eating but that are potentially deleterious to your health. Do not use butter for cooking; use olive oil or safflower oil instead. Use skim milk or 1-percent milk instead of whole milk or 2-percent milk. Use low-fat cottage cheese and yogurt. Use evaporated milk in recipes calling for heavy cream. Use low-fat yogurt in your dips and salad dressings instead of sour cream. It is recommended that you have at least two servings of 1-percent low-fat milk daily to maintain calcium intake.

### *Fats and Oils*

You will want to reduce the intake of fats and oils high in saturated fatty acids. Avoid butter, lard, beef fat, coconut oil, palm oil, and palm kernel oil. Read food labels carefully to make sure they do not contain these products, which are extremely high in saturated fatty acids.

Unsaturated vegetable oils—corn, cottonseed, safflower, soybean, sunflower—are acceptable when no more than 6 to 8 teaspoons are used per day. Since these oils are high in calories, their intake should be limited. See *The Barbara Kraus Calorie Counter* for exact amounts.

Although margarine and vegetable shortening contain partially hydrogenated vegetable oil, they are preferable to butter when taken in limited amounts.

## Breads, Cereals, Pasta, Rice, Dried Peas and Beans

Generally these products are low in fat and high in carbohydrates and protein. It is a good idea to substitute them for fatty foods. Use large quantities of whole grain pasta, brown rice, legumes, and vegetables with increasingly smaller amounts of lean meat, fish, or poultry to get complete protein with less fat, cholesterol, and calories.

Processed wheat products and processed flour should be avoided even if your cholesterol falls in the desirable range. It makes no sense to eat a product from which the nutritional value has already been extracted. Use whole grain breads, cereals with no salt or sugar added, and brown rice. High-fiber cereals eaten on a routine basis will guarantee benefits if you are meeting the minimum 10-to-20-gram daily requirement.

## Nuts

Nuts are high in unsaturated fatty acids and caloric value, but eaten in controlled amounts they are a good source of plant protein.

## Sauces and Gravies

Avoid rich, creamy sauces in general!

### *Chocolate*

Chocolate is high in saturated fat and should not be eaten often.

### *Alcohol and Coffee*

Curtail your intake of alcohol to no more than 2 ounces per day (8 ounces if wine). To consume more than that will elevate your simple sugars and triglycerides.

Scientific evidence indicates that excessive coffee drinking exacerbates cholesterol levels. Any stimulant can ultimately result in a heart problem.

Caffeine—a potent cardiovascular stimulator—affects the central nervous system, the peripheral nervous system, and the kidneys. It is a chemical as deleterious as nicotine and should be avoided. If you must drink coffee, drink decaffeinated coffee.

### *Poultry*

Chicken and turkey are high in protein. When you prepare poultry at home, remove the skin and clean away the underlying layers of fat before cooking. When you are dining out, remove the skin before eating. Avoid fried chicken and entrees prepared in rich, creamy sauces. Tomato and wine sauces are acceptable.

Poultry is a secondary source of calcium, but you must watch for its fat content. Unless you buy organically grown chicken without additives (much commercially prepared chicken has them), and unless you are very meticulous about how your chicken is prepared, if you overconsume even chicken you are doing yourself a disservice. Additionally, the infection rate in chickens is high from salmonella, a bacteria that infects the intestines and causes dysentery.

### *Fish and Fish Oils*

The omega 3 fish oils should be ingested in their organic state. There have been anecdotal reports of significant side effects associated with taking fish oils in capsule form: It depresses the immune system and can cause hemorrhages. In addition, there has been no benefit demonstrated in the lowering of triglycerides by high-dosage ingestion of these oils in a nonorganic fashion.

Fish—tuna, salmon, swordfish, scallops, halibut—is a fine source of protein. Again, preparation is important. You will want to avoid rich sauces. Marinate your fish in lemon, lime, tomato sauce, wine, onions, garlic, and your favorite herbs and spices and bake, broil, or steam it. (Steamed fish is a favorite breakfast food in the Bahamas!) Don't forget that most of the fat content of fish products is polyunsaturated, therefore you will want to eat fish often.

The problem of pollution of our waters increases daily with all kinds of waste and toxins washing ashore. You will need to be careful to select fresh fish from waters known to be safe.

### *Shellfish*

Lobster, shrimp, crabs, and other shellfish are regarded as the "red meat" of the sea. Because they are high in saturated fat, eat them on a very moderate basis, carefully measuring the amount of cholesterol and saturated fat in terms of the meal plan for the day.

You will need to reduce your intake of lean meat, chicken, turkey, and fish until you are eating no more than the recommended six ounces per day.

### Fruits and Vegetables

Fruit, an excellent source of dietary fiber, makes an excellent breakfast, snack, lunch, and dessert. Eat a wide variety of fresh raw fruit. Fruit is also a good source of B vitamins, vitamin C, and iron.

Eat a wide variety of raw or lightly steamed fresh vegetables daily.

### Desserts

Eat fruit, low-fat yogurt and fruit, fruit ices, sherbet, and angel food cake (the latter should be eaten in moderation due to its high calorie content).

### Eating Out

Avoid butter, large portions of untrimmed red meat, entrees prepared in sauces and gravies, and poultry with skin. Ask for margarine instead of butter and choose salads. But watch those salad dressings for fat content!

## THE PROGRAM FOR 20- TO 40-YEAR-OLDS

### 200–240 mg/dl (borderline high cholesterol)

Begin the program with the immediate cessation of cigarette smoking and the adoption of a regular exercise regimen.

If you are in this age range, if your blood lipid profile is in the borderline high range, and if you have fewer than two risk factors (refer to the list on page 25), dietary modification is the way to go. Drugs should not be considered in this range if you are risk factor deficient. You are young enough to develop lifelong patterns of healthy eating. After consultation with your doctor and a registered nutritionist, begin the Step-One Diet.

Follow the Step-One Diet for six months to a year, with close regular checking from your nutritionist that you are following the plan sufficiently to attain desirable cholesterol levels. Meet with your nutritionist at the end of the first six weeks to evaluate your progress. Consult with your nutritionist again at the end of three months and meet with your physician after this consultation. At that point your physician should do a nonfasting cholesterol test to see how effective your dietary manipulations have been.

If your physician is satisfied with your results, continue the diet, meeting with your nutritionist quarterly during the first year and semiannually thereafter to evaluate your adherence. See your doctor on a yearly basis for an examination of your lipid profile.

However, if at the end of three months your results are insubstantial, go back to your nutritionist for additional reinforcement. After three months of strict adherence that is corroborated by your nutritionist's evaluation, have yourself retested. If your adherence has not been sufficient to get the desired results, you should continue on the Step-One Diet until your adherence is satisfactory. If you are having trouble sticking to the diet and have not joined a support group, do so at once.

If your adherence to the Step-One Diet has been appropriate and at the end of three months there is little or no fall in your blood fats, go on to the Step-Two Diet. If at the end of six months on the Step-Two Diet you still have little or no fall in your lipid levels, your doctor might consider the use of niacin.

### *Over 240 total cholesterol*

If you are between 30 and 40 and your serum cholesterol is elevated above 240 mg/dl, you must aggressively manage your diet by weight loss and strict adherence to the Step-One

Diet. Consult your physician and nutritionist for assistance in daily meal planning, monitoring, and follow-up. In accordance with the recommendations of the Expert Panel on Detection, Evaluation, and Treatment of High Blood Cholesterol in Adults, if after three months you have not experienced an adequate fall in your cholesterol, after consultation with your physician and nutritionist you might proceed to the more restrictive Step-Two Diet. If adherence is the problem, you should stay on the Step-One Diet until proper adherence is achieved.

If your follow-up visits demonstrate strict adherence to the Step-One Diet and adequate drops in your blood fat totals, remain on the diet until you have achieved desirable levels.

However, if after strict adherence corroborated by the dietitian's evaluations, you have experienced no substantial fall in your cholesterol totals, after six months of strict adherence to both diets you will need to consider at least niacin as a drug, depending on the level of your triglycerides. Of course, this decision must be made in consultation with your physician and professional health team.

If you are between 20 and 40, have borderline totals between 200 and 240, but possess two or more risk factors, you will need to aggressively manage your adherence to the Step-One Diet. After three months if you have not experienced sufficient reductions in your blood fats, proceed immediately to the Step-Two Diet. Again, strict adherence is crucial. If at the end of six months of strict adherence on both diets you do not see adequate decreases, you will need to consider medication. Niacin is the drug of first choice. All drug therapy should be administered under the strict supervision of a physician who has experience with cholesterol management and is aware of the latest research data on diet and drugs.

If you are in this age range, possess two or more risk factors, and your elevation is above 240, you must strictly adhere to the program. If strict adherence is substantiated and your lipid profile shows no significant drop, go immediately to the Step-Two Diet. By the end of three months, if you have experienced no substantial fall, medication will probably be required.

Dietary modification, risk factor modification, and regular aerobic exercise are the trio of components of your cholesterol-lowering program. As you initiate dietary changes you should also begin a pattern of regular aerobic exercise. Your goal is to develop health-promoting habits and patterns that are lifelong.

If you smoke cigarettes, stop immediately. (Recommendations for doing this have been presented in an earlier chapter.) If you are overweight, reduce your caloric intake to bring your body weight to within 10 percent of your ideal weight.

If your total cholesterol is 240 and above and you are risk factor deficient, with an HDL in the range of 35 mg/dl or above, despite your elevated cholesterol you are considered to have one less risk factor.

## *THE PROGRAM FOR 40- TO 65-YEAR-OLDS*

If you are between these ages, you should pay close attention to your serum cholesterol levels. This is the middle-aged population especially prone to sudden cardiac death and to silent heart attacks. Symptoms cannot be your guide; one must use risk factor analysis to determine the aggressiveness of the treatment if your serum cholesterol is elevated. Your goal must be to bring your total cholesterol down to the 200 range or less. You must do this aggressively. Remember, you are in the group most prone to coronary risk. This is especially true of men in this age range with two or more risk factors.

### *200–240 mg/dl (borderline high cholesterol)*

It is of the utmost necessity that you adhere to the Step-One Diet. If after three months you experience no substantial fall, go immediately to the Step-Two Diet and observe strict adherence. It is very important that you do not rely on the appearance of symptoms to initiate and follow a strict dietary regimen if you are in this group—20 to 30 percent of all attacks of greatest risk that occur in the middle-aged population occur totally silently, without any symptoms whatsoever, and are discovered retrospectively on routine tests by electrocardiology. You should undergo screening procedures on a yearly basis that search for the presence of asymptomatic disease. You also need a yearly stress test to see if you have developed any significant diagnostic changes in your EKG at peak exercise levels.

### *Over 240 total cholesterol*

If you are between 40 and 65 years of age, your total cholesterol is 241 or over, and you have fewer than two coronary risk factors, your condition demands aggressive management of your cholesterol totals. You will want to aggressively lower your cholesterol because of the possibility of accumulated damage that has already occurred. Within the first six months, with assurance that you have been following the sequential Step-One and Step-Two diets without substantial lowering of your cholesterol total, your physician may very well consider medication.

If your LDL level is above 225 mg/dl, your physician may consider instituting diet and drug therapy nearly simultaneously, certainly within six weeks if there has been no appreciable fall in your levels and it is verified that you have strictly followed the daily meal plan. The risk for a coronary event at these levels is quite high. For each point of cholesterol elevation above 240, the degree of risk for coronary disease begins to increase in an exponential fashion. Bear in mind that it is the *accumulated* effect that is so dangerous.

To insure satisfactory adherence, obtain regular feedback from your physician on your cholesterol levels. Devise a self-monitoring system with your physician's support. Maintain regularly scheduled follow-up with your physician and nutritionist. When you are undergoing periods of stress or change, increase the frequency of your telephone and personal contact with your physician and nutritionist.

## THE PROGRAM FOR 65-YEAR-OLDS AND BEYOND

### 200–240 mg/dl (borderline high cholesterol)

In the elderly person dietary restrictions must be balanced against the possibility of inadequate or inappropriate nutrition. The Step-One Diet, after consultation with your doctor, may be advisable. Usually restrictions greater than that are not advisable. If you have not had a coronary attack prior to age 65, it has not been medically established that aggressive management of hyperlipidemia at that age will necessarily prevent one.

### Over 240 total cholesterol

If you are physiologically young despite your age and have elevated cholesterol above 240, you may wish to manage it aggressively. In general, elderly people should consult with their physicians about the appropriate means for management of their blood lipid profile.

A well-structured diet that is moderate in its fat and cholesterol intake can only be beneficial. It will help keep the tendency to excessive weight in check. In fact, it just makes good overall sense and certainly does promote good overall health in children, adults, and older people to follow a diet that is structured along the lines of the Step-One Diet.

Do not underestimate the importance of exercise even at 65 and beyond. Aerobic exercise alone can produce a 10-percent fall in your blood lipid levels. It is an important component of the cholesterol-lowering program presented here. The success of your cholesterol program will depend almost entirely upon your adherence to dietary restriction, regular exercise, and risk modification. If medication becomes necessary, your strict adherence to that schedule is also fundamental to good results.

Again we say: Low fat, high fiber, and regular aerobic exercise are *pro* life!

# 4
# Healthy Eating Habits

Cutting dietary cholesterol is clearly vital to good health, and the most effective strategy for doing so is to decrease the amount of saturated fat consumed daily since it is the main culprit in high blood lipid profiles. The cholesterol intake recommended by the American Heart Association is not to exceed 300 mg per day. On a traditional high-fat diet, you can hit that limit by the time you finish breakfast! Don't be discouraged, however. You can still eat a varied and appetizing diet when armed with the proper information and a little imagination.

A modest reduction in consumption of egg yolks and organ meats can lower blood cholesterol levels slightly; concentrated, daily dietary modification can result in significant reduction in your lipid levels, particularly when accompanied by regular aerobic exercise. Adjusting your lifestyle and eating habits to lower your cholesterol will help you to live longer and healthier.

The menus that follow are samples to get you started. They should be adjusted to meet with the requirements of the diet your physician has placed you on in terms of calories, saturated fat, cholesterol, sugar, and sodium. As a general rule, it is always best to avoid simple sugars and to select low-sodium products.

All of the bread, pasta, and cereal products included in the menus are made with whole grains, without egg yolks (or fall in the allowable amount of saturated fat for the day), and with low-fat milk and the proper vegetable oils. All milk products are of the low-fat variety. For salads, use dressings made with the allowable oils and/or low-fat ingredients.

When preparing beans it is best to use dried or fresh varieties. If you are using dried beans such as pintos, navy beans, or black-eyed peas, wash and soak them for 6 to 8 hours before cooking. Soaking enhances the flavor, shortens the cooking time, and reduces gases in dried beans and peas.

The menus promote the use of polyunsaturated fat to help reduce cholesterol. They de-emphasize the use of animal products, which are high in both saturated fat and cholesterol, while emphasizing tasty, appealing entrees.

When buying beef, select only lean, well-trimmed cuts. Since the "Prime" graded meats are highly marbled, they contain more fat; buy "Choice" and "Good" graded meat instead. If your doctor has placed you on a very strict caloric regimen and you must weigh your meat, remove all bones and skin before weighing the cooked portion. Limit your intake to no more than 6 ounces daily.

Although you will not find them listed on the menus below, soybeans and soybean products are excellent sources of protein. When using soy products, read the label to ascertain that no saturated fat has been added.

You may eat egg whites freely, but you must limit your intake of egg yolks to 2 or less per week. Try to keep your intake of egg yolk to 1 per week. Since it will be difficult to count exact measures of egg yolks used in cooking and in baking breads and cakes, watch your consumption of these food items. Avoid cakes, cookies, mixes, and other commercial foods containing egg yolks.

Avoid imitation sour creams, coffee creamers, filled milk, imitation milk, and processed foods in general. You will notice that the items included on the menu lists are nearly always fresh, whole products.

Consume raw vegetables and fruits daily. An excellent way to get a zestful, refreshing, low-calorie drink full of vitamins, minerals, and nutrients is to have several glasses of fresh-squeezed fruit and vegetable juices daily. It is also important that you drink several glasses of water every day. Ideally you should consume 6 to 8 glasses of liquid each day.

Augment your intake of carbohydrates by including starchy vegetables such as yellow and green squash, winter squash, beans, hominy, sweet potatoes, white potatoes, and pumpkin in your meals often.

Soups are an excellent source of nutrition and make very tasty meals. You may freely use fat-free broth, bouillon, consommé, and creamed soups made with low-fat milk. When making beef stew, cut down on the number of beef chunks used and increase the number of chunks of potatoes, eggplant, zucchini, and carrots; remove all excess fat before serving. Tofu makes an excellent filler for stew. If you are preparing a tuna dish, use only the water-packed variety.

You will need to limit the amounts of margarine, nuts, oils, and seeds according to the caloric intake of your plan. Salads, soups, and casseroles are excellent when garnished with sunflower seeds, almonds, or walnuts.

Add zest and nutrition to your salads by garnishing them liberally with alfalfa, bean, radish, and other sprouts.

Whenever possible it is best to plan your meals in advance. This will help you in shopping and in preparing portions that allow you to stay within the limits of your new dietary program. It also will allow you to consult your Barbara Kraus cholesterol and calorie counters before you sit down to eat. And if you are contemplating selecting unfamiliar items when you are eating out, consult the counters as well. After a while you will become familiar with the proportions allowed for the foods you eat most often.

Attention to good food-combining practices and good taste as well as to the ratios of saturated fats to unsaturated fats and fatty acids to total calories underlies the creation of the menus presented here for breakfast, lunch, dinner, and snacks. Adjust the menus according to your needs and taste. They are provided to help you adhere to the Step-One and/or Step-Two dietary regimen for the first month. They are also provided to demonstrate that you can eat a wide variety of food and still adhere to the diet.

Your portions should comply with the guidelines of the diet. Whether you are on the Step-One or Step-Two diet, you should keep your total caloric intake at a level that will allow you to achieve and maintain a desirable weight. Carbohydrates should comprise at least 50 percent of your total calories, with protein comprising no more than 20 percent. As you use these menus and prepare your meals, you should also keep total fat intake (saturated, polyunsaturated, and monounsaturated fatty acids) within the recommended limits outlined in the Step-One and Step-Two diets.

The menus that follow are models of what you can do, and are provided to get you started. Use them until you feel comfortable creating your own plan. Again, it is important to plan ahead. Choose menus one week at a time, then shop according to a prepared grocery list that includes staples such as brown rice, beans, pasta, tomato sauce, potatoes, and onions. Plan several shopping trips to allow for ample time to compare prices and read labels. Visit your local health food store, where you will find a wide variety of low-fat items and whole grain products. When it comes to seafood and to fresh vegetables and fruits, it is not desirable to buy ahead more than two or three days. These items are best when served fresh.

It is of enormous importance to remember that the menus provided here are a guide merely for the *first* 30 days on your cholesterol-lowering diet. This is not a temporary diet, something you go on or off as you want to shed a few pounds or take a few inches off your waist or thighs. This will be a *permanent* change in your eating habits.

It is this primary strategy that must guide you daily as you attempt to carry out the Step-One or Step-Two diet along with exercise and risk modification. Begin to cook and serve smaller portions of meat while offering generous servings of mixed vegetable salads, potatoes, brown rice, pasta, wheat pilaf, baked squash, green vegetables, low-fat soups, and whole grain breads. You will want to cook and serve red meat with decreasing frequency until you are eating and serving it no more than once a week. Begin to substitute skinless poultry and fish entrees for red meat. Rock Cornish hen or Norwegian salmon are delicious, healthy substitutes for steak or roast beef.

When it comes to fish it is hard to go wrong. A serving of fish is lower in saturated fat than skinned chicken and it contains about half the cholesterol. Tuna, mackerel, salmon, and herring are very good selections since they have higher concentrations of the polyunsaturated omega 3 fatty acids that are reported to protect against atherosclerosis and some forms of cancer. On the other hand, you will want to watch your consumption of shellfish such as shrimp and lobster since they have high cholesterol contents. It is a good idea to eat these seafoods seldom and to limit your portion to 3 ounces.

If you are on a weight-loss diet as well as a cholesterol-lowering program, it is best to keep your use of unsaturated oils to 6 to 8 teaspoons per day because of their generally high calorie content.

By determination, discipline, and consistency, you can lower your intake of fatty acids and cholesterol, decrease your risk for coronary heart disease, shed unnecessary body fat, and still eat a wide variety of good-tasting food.

Remember: Low fat and high fiber are *pro* life!

## *MENUS FOR 30 DAYS*

### Day 1

**BREAKFAST**

orange juice (fresh-squeezed preferred)
banana
homemade granola cereal
skim or soy milk with honey
whole wheat toast with margarine

**LUNCH**

apple juice
vegetarian chili
lettuce and tomato salad
toasted tortilla chips
oat bran muffins

**SNACK**

apple

**DINNER**

broiled red snapper in lemon sauce
brown rice
steamed broccoli
mixed vegetable salad with low-fat yogurt dressing
whole wheat Italian bread
margarine
angel food cake

### Day 2

**BREAKFAST**

cantaloupe
oat bran muffins
margarine
skim milk

**LUNCH**

tuna sandwich (water-packed)
mayonnaise
whole grain bread
raw veggies
grape juice
frozen fruit bar

**SNACK**

large pear

**DINNER**

medley of vegetable salad with Italian dressing
baked chicken (skinned)
acorn squash
sourdough bread
gelatin with fruit

**SNACK**

carrot sticks

## Day 3

**BREAKFAST**

apple juice
oat bran cereal with skim or soy milk and honey or molasses
whole wheat toast with margarine

**LUNCH**

turkey sandwich (skinned) with mayonnaise, lettuce, tomato, and pickles
artichoke hearts and carrot sticks
skim milk
oat bran muffins with raisins

**SNACK**

grapes

**DINNER**

chopped vegetable mélange sautéed in olive oil
brown rice garnished with walnuts
cucumber salad
pita bread
iced tea
sherbet

**SNACK**

lightly salted air-popped popcorn (no butter)

## Day 4

**BREAKFAST**

orange juice
oatmeal with raisins, evaporated skim milk, and honey or brown sugar
rye toast with margarine
banana

**LUNCH**

lettuce and tomato salad with lemon juice and herbs
ratatouille
French bread with margarine
grape juice
frozen yogurt

**SNACK**

trail mix

**DINNER**

baked salmon in lemon herb sauce
carrots and green peas
baked potato with margarine and onion powder
pumpernickel bread
coleslaw
fruit ice

**SNACK**

grapes

## Day 5

**BREAKFAST**

- grapefruit
- shredded wheat with strawberries and skim milk
- whole wheat bagel with margarine
- decaffeinated coffee or tea

**LUNCH**

- mixed vegetable salad with Italian dressing
- chicken cacciatore with spaghetti
- whole grain roll
- skim milk
- fruit cup

**SNACK**

- raisins

**DINNER**

- broiled T-bone steak (lean and well trimmed "Choice" or "Good" grades)
- three bean salad
- steamed broccoli and whole mushrooms with margarine
- garlic bread
- angel food cake

**SNACK**

- rye crisp

## Day 6

**BREAKFAST**

- oat bran cereal with skim or soy milk, chopped apple, and honey
- whole wheat toast with margarine
- orange juice
- decaffeinated coffee or tea

**LUNCH**

- vegetable soup
- tossed salad with lemon juice
- boiled egg
- rye bread
- oat bran muffin made with fruit

**SNACK**

- pear

**DINNER**

- baked trout in lemon herb mustard sauce
- wild rice
- asparagus
- mixed vegetable salad with Russian dressing
- whole wheat dinner rolls
- margarine
- sherbet

**SNACK**

- air-popped popcorn (no butter)

## Day 7

**BREAKFAST**

date bran muffin
grapefruit juice
ham (center slice, rump, or shank)
skim milk

**LUNCH**

peanut butter sandwich on whole grain bread
apple sauce
raw veggies
skim milk
frozen fruit bar

**SNACK**

melba toast and carrot sticks

**DINNER**

spinach pasta with seafood tomato sauce
tossed salad with vinegar and oil
steamed cauliflower
sherbet

**SNACK**

graham crackers and fresh strawberries

## Day 8

**BREAKFAST**

grapefruit
scrambled egg whites in safflower oil
raisin bread toast
decaffeinated coffee or tea

**LUNCH**

pinto beans and brown rice
raw veggies
jalapeño cornbread
lettuce and tomato salad with French dressing

**SNACK**

peach

**DINNER**

grilled salmon steak
baked potato
zucchini
carrot salad
hard roll

**SNACK**

air-popped popcorn (no butter)

## Day 9

**BREAKFAST**

orange juice
oatmeal with sliced banana
whole wheat English muffin with margarine
decaffeinated coffee or tea

**LUNCH**

hamburger (lean and well-trimmed chuck or round)
tossed salad with lemon juice
frozen fruit bar
iced tea

**DINNER**

vegetable salad medley with yogurt dressing
baked turkey
stuffed pepper (tomato and brown rice)
sweet potato
angel food cake

**SNACK**

melba toast

## Day 10

**BREAKFAST**

orange juice
oat bran muffins with dates
banana
skim milk

**LUNCH**

lentil soup
avocado salad with sprouts and lemon herb dressing
pumpernickel bread with margarine

**DINNER**

tossed salad with alfalfa sprouts and Italian dressing
consommé (fat-free) with rye crisp
baked red snapper marinated in lemon, garlic, onions, and herbs
spinach fettuccine in marinara sauce
whole grain bread
yogurt and fruit

**SNACK**

saltines

## Day 11

**BREAKFAST**

pineapple juice
Wheatena with evaporated skim milk and honey
English muffin with margarine
banana

**LUNCH**

vegetarian pizza
lettuce and tomato salad with lemon juice
ginger ale (low-calorie)
frozen fruit bar

**SNACK**

raw veggies

**DINNER**

veal cutlet
mashed potatoes with skim milk and margarine
steamed spinach
dinner roll
coleslaw with tomato slices

**SNACK**

graham crackers

## Day 12

**BREAKFAST**

pineapple juice
Grape-Nuts cereal with skim or soy milk, honey, and raisins
English muffin
boiled egg

**LUNCH**

lentil soup and saltines
tuna sandwich (water-packed) with mayonnaise, lettuce, and tomato on rye bread
raw veggies
cranapple juice

**SNACK**

pear

**DINNER**

barbecued chicken
Spanish rice
mixed vegetable salad with sprouts and French dressing
whole wheat oatmeal bread
French-style green beans
margarine
gelatin

**SNACK**

pretzels

## Day 13

**BREAKFAST**

grape juice
whole wheat pancakes
maple syrup
low-fat yogurt and fresh peaches

**LUNCH**

fresh fruit salad with low-fat yogurt, honey, and nuts
oat bran muffins

**SNACK**

dried fruit and nuts

**DINNER**

tuna and whole grain macaroni casserole
carrot raisin salad
acorn squash
steamed broccoli
dinner roll
lime sherbet

**SNACK**

grapes

## Day 14

**BREAKFAST**

orange juice
oat bran cereal with skim or soy milk and honey
scrambled egg whites
whole wheat bagel

**LUNCH**

minestrone soup
melba toast
cheese sandwich on pumpernickel toast with lettuce and tomatoes
frozen fruit bar

**SNACK**

trail mix

**DINNER**

vegetable lasagna
steamed cauliflower
French bread
tossed salad with Italian dressing
angel food cake

**SNACK**

air-popped popcorn (no butter)

## Day 15

**BREAKFAST**

apple juice
French toast (made with whole wheat bread, egg, and skim milk; honey, jelly, or light syrup topping)

**LUNCH**

turkey sandwich on whole wheat with mustard, lettuce, tomato
raw veggies
split pea soup
saltines
fruit-filled oat bran muffins

**SNACK**

oat bran muffins

**DINNER**

broiled lamb chops (lean and well trimmed)
baked potato with margarine and onion powder
fresh lima beans
lettuce and tomato salad with lemon juice and herbs

**SNACK**

papaya

## Day 16

**BREAKFAST**

tomato juice
cold cereal with skim milk
banana nut bread
boiled egg

**LUNCH**

Waldorf salad
ratatouille
oat bran muffins

**SNACK**

apple

**DINNER**

broiled sea bass in lemon/tomato sauce
whole grain pasta
sautéed mushrooms and eggplant
mixed vegetable salad
sherbet

**SNACK**

rye crisp

## Day 17

**BREAKFAST**
orange juice
scrambled egg whites
oat bran muffins
skim milk

**LUNCH**
vegetarian chili with beans
low-fat cheese
bread sticks
raw veggies
frozen fruit bar

**SNACK**
oat bran muffin

**DINNER**
gazpacho
Cornish hen
steamed zucchini
brown rice
mixed vegetable salad

**SNACK**
apple

## Day 18

**BREAKFAST**
poached egg
cranapple juice
toasted raisin bread
skim milk

**LUNCH**
chicken cutlet sandwich on pumpernickel with mayonnaise, lettuce, tomato
crudité salad
fresh fruit cup

**DINNER**
vichyssoise
broiled filet of sole in lemon herb sauce
brown and wild rice mix
Brussels sprouts and carrots
tossed salad
sourdough bread
strawberries and low-fat yogurt

**SNACK**
homemade granola

## Day 19

**BREAKFAST**
- oatmeal with sliced apples, honey, and skim evaporated milk
- banana nut bread
- orange juice

**LUNCH**
- vegetable soup
- pasta with marinara sauce
- lettuce and tomato salad
- melba toast
- frozen yogurt

**SNACK**
- apple

**DINNER**
- Hawaiian chicken
- potato salad garnished with fresh sliced tomato and parsley
- corn on the cob
- whole wheat rolls
- orange sherbet

**SNACK**
- graham crackers

## Day 20

**BREAKFAST**
- orange juice
- banana
- oat bran muffins
- skim milk

**LUNCH**
- shrimp gumbo
- lettuce and tomato salad
- oyster crackers
- seedless grapes

**SNACK**
- graham crackers

**DINNER**
- poached salmon
- whole wheat spaghetti with tomato sauce
- mixed vegetable salad
- green peas
- hard roll
- fruit ice
- iced tea

**SNACK**
- bread sticks

## Day 21

**BREAKFAST**
- tomato juice
- oat bran cereal with raisins, skim milk, and honey
- whole wheat toast
- decaffeinated coffee or tea

**LUNCH**
- cranapple juice
- peanut butter sandwich on whole wheat toast
- fruit salad
- sherbet

**SNACK**
- trail mix

**DINNER**
- roast beef
- mashed potatoes with margarine and skim milk
- steamed cabbage
- lettuce and tomato salad with lemon juice and basil
- garlic bread
- gelatin

**SNACK**
- bread sticks

## Day 22

**BREAKFAST**
- orange juice
- granola
- oat bran muffins
- skim milk

**LUNCH**
- cranapple juice
- chicken rice soup
- oyster crackers
- lettuce and tomato salad with French dressing
- frozen fruit bar

**SNACK**
- pear

**DINNER**
- broiled bluefish
- Spanish rice
- asparagus spears
- three bean salad
- monk bread
- raspberry sherbet

**SNACK**
- air-popped popcorn

## Day 23

**BREAKFAST**

orange juice
boiled egg
oat bran muffins
decaffeinated coffee or tea

**LUNCH**

tomato juice
turkey sandwich on rye with mayonnaise, lettuce, and tomato
barley soup
skim milk
pear

**SNACK**

nuts and raisins

**DINNER**

baked chicken
wild rice
steamed broccoli
lettuce and tomato salad with lemon juice and herbs
French bread
angel food cake
iced tea

**SNACK**

graham crackers

## Day 24

**BREAKFAST**

assorted fresh fruit
oat bran muffins
skim milk

**LUNCH**

tuna and assorted raw veggies in whole wheat pita bread
fresh strawberries
date bran muffin

**SNACK**

grapes

**DINNER**

vegetarian chili
brown rice
raw veggies
avocado salad with lemon juice and thyme
oatmeal bread
fresh fruit

**SNACK**

bread sticks

## Day 25

**BREAKFAST**
- grapefruit
- cold cereal with skim milk and honey
- whole wheat bagel and low-fat cream cheese
- decaffeinated coffee or tea

**LUNCH**
- split pea soup
- lettuce and tomato salad
- melba toast
- pear

**SNACK**
- raisins

**DINNER**
- baked halibut in wine sauce
- baked potato with margarine
- heart of palm salad with tomato slices
- steamed zucchini strips
- ice milk

**SNACK**
- air-popped popcorn

## Day 26

**BREAKFAST**
- pineapple juice
- baked apple
- oat bran muffins
- skim milk

**LUNCH**
- corn chowder
- curry chicken
- mixed green salad with Italian dressing
- bread sticks
- frozen fruit bar

**SNACK**
- apple

**DINNER**
- baked turkey
- mashed potatoes
- French green beans
- mixed vegetable salad
- dinner roll
- gelatin

**SNACK**
- graham crackers

## Day 27

**BREAKFAST**

oat bran cereal with skim milk, raisins, and honey
oat bran muffins with dates
orange juice

**LUNCH**

mushroom soup
carrot and celery sticks
English muffin with fruit spread
fresh fruit cup

**SNACK**

raisins and nuts

**DINNER**

veal scaloppine
linguine with tomato sauce
spinach
mixed green salad with French dressing
Italian bread
sherbet

**SNACK**

rye crisp

## Day 28

**BREAKFAST**

pancakes and light syrup
orange juice
fresh blueberries and low-fat yogurt

**LUNCH**

Low-fat cottage cheese and fresh fruit salad
minestrone soup
oat bran muffins
frozen fruit bar

**SNACK**

apple

**DINNER**

baked salmon
sautéed eggplant, mushrooms, and fresh tomatoes with basil
baked potato
avocado salad with picante sauce
angel food cake

**SNACK**

carrot sticks

## Day 29

**BREAKFAST**

tomato juice
ham (very thinly sliced)
oat bran muffins

**LUNCH**

tuna sandwich on whole wheat with lettuce and tomato
raw veggies
potato salad
Jell-O
iced tea

**SNACK**

raisins and nuts

**DINNER**

barbecued chicken
pasta salad
coleslaw
green beans
dinner roll
sherbet

**SNACK**

air-popped popcorn

## Day 30

**BREAKFAST**

cold cereal with skim milk
banana
orange juice
bagel

**LUNCH**

ratatouille
mixed green salad
hard roll
apple

**SNACK**

frozen fruit bar

**DINNER**

hearty beef stew with eggplant chunks
green beans
mixed green salad with lemon juice and herbs
gelatin

**SNACK**

bread sticks

# A QUICK-REFERENCE FOOD LIST

## *FOODS TO EAT FREELY*

### BEVERAGES

decaffeinated coffee
decaffeinated tea
skim milk
skim buttermilk
skim evaporated milk
all fruit and vegetable juices
carbonated drinks

### FRUIT

apples, *seb*
apricots, *khubani*
bananas, *kela*
blackberries, *jamun*
blueberries, *neelbadri*
cantaloupes, *kharbuza*
cranberries, *karonda*
dates, *khajur*
figs, *anjeer*
grapefruits, *chakotra*
grapes, *angoor*
mangoes, *aam*
nectarines, *shattalu*
oranges, *santara*
papayas, *papita*
peaches, *aaru*
pears, *nashpati*
pineapples, *ananas*
plums, *alu bukhara*
prunes, *aloocha*
raisins, *munaqqa*
raspberries, *rasbhari*
strawberries, *hisalu*
tangerines, *santara*
watermelon, *tarbuz*

### VEGETABLES

alfalfa sprouts, *ankurit rijka*
artichokes, *hathichak*
asparagus, *shatwari*,
  *soot mooli, halyan*
bamboo shoots, *baans ka ankur*
bean sprouts, *phallion ka ankur*
beans, *phalliyan*
beets, *chukandar*
broccoli, *phulgobhi*
Brussels sprouts, *bandhgobhi*
  *ka guda*
cabbage, *bandgobhi*
cauliflower, *phulgobhi*
celery, *ajmod*
cucumbers, *khira*
eggplant, *baigan*
endive, *kasani*
escarole, endive plant leaves
ginger, *adrak*
greens
  beet, *chukander*
  collard
  dandelion
  kale, *karamsaag*
  mustard, *rai, sarson*
  spinach, *palak*
  Swiss chard
  turnip, *shalgam*
lettuce, *salad patta*
mushrooms, *khombi*
okra, *bhindi*
onions, *piyaz*
parsley, *ajmod*
peppers, *mirch*

potatoes, *alu, ratalu*
pumpkin, *kashiphal*
radishes, *muli*
sauerkraut, *shakarkand*
sprouts, *ankur*
squash, *sharbet*
  acorn, *banjuphal, banjphul*
  butternut, *amriki akhrot*
  spaghetti
  zucchini
tomatoes, *tamatar*
turnips, *shalgam*
watercress, *jalkhumbi*

FISH

all salt- and fresh-water varieties

BREAD AND CRACKERS

whole grain breads
whole grain pasta
bread sticks
graham crackers
matzo
melba toast
biscuits
noodles
cornflakes

DESSERTS

fruit ice
gelatin
sherbet

CEREAL

oat bran, *jaunka atta*
wheat bran, *gehun ka atta*
oatmeal, *jaun ka dalia*
rice

DAIRY

egg whites

***FOODS TO EAT MODERATELY***

DAIRY

low-fat yogurt, *dahi*
low-fat cheese, *paneer*
skim chocolate milk

FRUIT

avocado, *kulu naspati,*

MEAT

lean meat
chicken (chest portion only)
beef (graded "Choice" or "Good"; lean and trimmed)
  chuck roast
  flank steak
  ground beef, *keema*
  porterhouse steak,
  sirloin steak, *puthe kaman*
  T-bone steak
  tenderloin, *mansal bhag*
  veal, *bachhara ka mans*
pork, *suar ka mans*
  center-cut ham slices
  leg
  loin
  ribs

SEAFOOD

crab, *kekra*
lobster, *ghinga*
shrimp, *chingat*

DESSERT

angel food cake

VEGETABLE OILS

corn oil, *makai ka tel*
olive oil, *jaitun ka tel*
safflower oil, *kusum, kusumbha*
sunflower oil, *suryamukhi ka tel*

**FOODS TO AVOID**

DAIRY

whole milk
chocoate milk
condensed milk
evaporated milk
malted milk
eggnog
egg yolks
butter
ice cream

COMMERCIALLY PREPARED FOODS

cakes
cookies
donuts
pancakes
pies
sweet rolls
waffles
frostings
fruit pie fillings
granola
simple sugars
whole milk cheese

VEGETABLE OILS

coconut oil, *nariyal ka tel*
palm oil, *tad ka tel*
palm kernel oil, *tad ke beej ka tel*

ANIMAL FAT

cream, *malai*
half-and-half
lard, *charbi*
shortening, *charbi*
sour cream, *makkhan*

FOOD SUBSTITUTES

nondairy cream substitutes
nondairy toppings

COMMERCIALLY FRIED FOODS

eggplant, *baigan*
french fries
okra, *bhindi*
onion rings
potatoes

MEAT

precooked canned and frozen meats
beef (graded "Prime")
- brains
- brisket, breast meat
- corned
- heart
- hot dogs
- liver
- lunch meat
- pastrami
- ribs
- rib eye

- sausage
- tongue

pork

- bacon
- Boston roast or steak
- cured ham
- ground
- ham hock
- neck bones
- picnic
- pigs' feet
- salt pork
- sausage
- spareribs

FISH AND POULTRY

caviar
duck
goose

BREAD AND SNACKS

all bread made with whole eggs
all pasta made with whole eggs
canned biscuits
cheesecake
cheese doodles
chocolate candy
corn chips
croissants
    bread roll
potato chips
tortilla chips
dry nuts

SAUCES

cheese sauces
cream sauces

OIL

hydrogenated oils

# 5
# The Importance of Aerobic Exercise

Aerobic is defined as living in, active in, or taking place in the presence of oxygen. Aerobic exercise refers to the endurance exercises that produce beneficial changes in our respiratory and circulatory systems by requiring only modest increases in our oxygen intake. This exercise includes such activities as walking, swimming, jogging, cycling, cross-country skiing, jumping rope, and aerobic dancing. When you are physically fit you can perform aerobic exercises for hours at a time and your breath will be regular, because you are using oxygen at about the same rate as you are taking it in and have no need to gasp for additional air.

Do not confuse aerobic exercise with anaerobic exercise, which causes your body to use more oxygen than you are taking in. As you push your body to its limits, your respiratory system is imbalanced and you become out of breath and exhausted. These exercises include activities such as sprinting and weight lifting.

Aerobic exercises are the most beneficial for weight loss, lowering your blood lipid levels, increasing your energy level, promoting your general well-being, and longevity. As you burn off excess body weight during exercise, your total cholesterol decreases. The aerobic effect allows you to achieve a high level of output at a low pulse rate.

An aerobically fit heart works much more efficiently; it does not require an increase in heart rate to increase its output as much as a deconditioned heart does. The so-called athlete's heart increases its output as the metabolic demands of the body rise by increasing its stroke volume, the amount of blood ejected with each beat. The highly conditioned heart does not have to increase the total heart rate—the number of beats per minute—to achieve an increase in output. Aerobic conditioning is reflected in the ability to sustain longer and longer periods of exercise to achieve increased heartbeat rates. It also results in a more rapid return of your accelerated heart rate to normal when exercise is discontinued. In your resting state you will notice your resting pulse gradually getting slower. This reflects the efficient working of your heart.

Aerobic exercise is the practice of repetitive flexing and retracting of muscle groups to bring about a gradual and predictable acceleration in heart rate. Aerobics is cardio-protective as opposed to isometrics, which is straining against a fixed resistance such as free weights or Nautilus resistance machines and is neither cardio-protective nor cardio-beneficial and does not increase endurance. When we recommend exercise, we are talking about pure aerobics. It is the aerobic phase of exercise that will protect against sudden cardiac death and hopefully lead to long life. A group of cardiologists and internists at the Mayo Clinic report that regular aerobic exercise of moderate duration—20 to 45 minutes, three to five times per week—has been shown to reduce serum triglycerides, to increase HDLs, and to have an overall beneficial effect on blood lipid profiles.

The regular practice of aerobic exercise is the most efficient method of caloric expenditure and is, therefore, beneficial for weight loss and reduction of stress. It tends to promote the general well-being of those who practice it. If you attempt dietary modification without aerobic exercise, you are cheating yourself. The benefit of any nutritional program is increased with regular exercise.

The benefits of aerobic exercise are multiple. Exercise happens to be one of the few inexpensive methods of stress reduction available. You can make it expensive, but one of the most beneficial aerobic exercises is walking. Walking at a brisk pace, a block or so per minute for a half mile to a mile three times a week—depending upon your endurance—will do you enormous good. If you are 20 or older, regular exercise is crucial to physical fitness. And physical fitness is crucial to long-lasting good health. But remember: Before beginning a program of exercise, consult your physician.

## GETTING STARTED

Your ability to withstand aerobic exercise depends on proper preparation and proper cool-down. You wouldn't think of walking out on a cold morning, getting into your car, turning the ignition, and driving off; you would let it warm up before pushing it into action. The same principle of caution should apply to your body machine. Before you begin any form of aerobic exercise, you will need to warm up by stretching for at least five minutes. The ability of your muscles, tendons, and joints to handle the stress of exercise is directly linked to stretching that occurs before and following the aerobic phase. Without adequate warm-up you may pull or tear tendons or muscles.

The most expensive health clubs in the world will teach you stretches that are merely variations of simple yoga positions. If you are about to begin an aerobic program, take a yoga class that is comfortable and conducted at a pace you can follow easily. In this atmosphere you will learn excellent stretching techniques, proper breathing, and proper relaxation techniques.

> *Stress is intimately linked to all of the diseases that are tied to heart disease, either as a major or minor determinant. The breathing exercises, stretching and relaxation techniques you learn in a real yoga class are very beneficial. Yoga is an ancient art form which has survived for thousands of years for a reason. It is highly effective, not expensive to learn and can be practiced by all.*
>
> —Dr. Alan Beckles

Use your newly learned yoga stretching techniques for several minutes before running, walking, swimming, jogging Use it following your aerobic workout to cool down. Never stop the concentrated phase of your exercise abruptly; it is extremely dangerous to do so. For at least 5 minutes following the concentrated phase, move around, gradually slowing down.

Don't forget: What you do after you finish the concentrated phase of aerobic exercise is as important as what you do before you begin. Adequate stretching before and after your concentrated phase of aerobic activity may prevent the development of problems in your back, upper body, or extremities.

A 59-year-old woman does yoga for half an hour every day and rides a stationary bicycle for half an hour three times a week to achieve physical fitness. This lady is in fantastic aerobic condition; has an amazing resting pulse in the high 40s, which is a direct benefit of her exercise program—and all accomplished in the familiar comfort of her home.

Not only is she in superb condition because of the bicycling and stretching that she does; she also has learned how to regulate her own resting pulse by breathing. Her resting pulse when she is not upset or stressed is extraordinarily slow. It is as slow as the pulse of most people when they are asleep.

Your aerobic exercise program should be tailored to your needs and enjoyment. It should be viewed as one very necessary component in your overall program to manage your blood lipids and more than likely prevent the development of artery-clogging atherosclerotic plaque and premature heart attack.

## Stress Testing

Stress testing is an effective screen for asymptomatic coronary heart disease. It is usually performed on a treadmill. After a series of electrocardiograms (EKGs) in various positions, you exercise on the treadmill, attempting to achieve a heart rate of 85 to 90 percent of the maximum predicted heart rate for your age. (See the formula on page 68.) If the test is to have diagnostic accuracy, that is the heart rate level that must be achieved.

An appropriate interpretation of the results of your stress test will rely on the principle of Bayes's theorem. Bayes's theorem states that the predictive accuracy of any noninvasive test depends upon the prevalency of the disease in the subpopulation being studied. So stress testing has the highest diagnostic accuracy in middle-aged men because they have the highest incidence of coronary heart disease in this country. A stress test must be interpreted in light of those limitations. In the population where the occurrence of CHD is the highest, the middle-aged male, the stress test has a diagnostic accuracy of 70 to 85 percent. This means that there is a 15 to 30 percent chance of false negative results. Any so-called normal stress test where there are no significant EKG changes must be interpreted with the statistical limitations of the test borne in mind.

Likewise, it is well known that women have a higher incidence of false positives when taking a stress test. When a woman uses the treadmill stress test, the results have even lower specificity. An abnormal stress test in a woman must be interpreted with that knowledge in mind.

The results of a negative stress test in men should be interpreted on the basis of the presence or absence of risk factors, not on the basis of the absence of symptoms. CHD is an asymptomatic disease and can progress to a massive heart attack without warning. Your concern is not the absence of symptoms, it is the presence of risk factors. Modern cardiovascular concepts place the attention on detecting an asymptomatic disease. A significant proportion of sudden cardiac death or first myocardial infarction comes without any warning at all. Often cardiac death—as much as two-thirds—is caused by a fatal rhythm disturbance, not by a fatal heart attack. Fatal rhythm disturbance, however, most often occurs in the presence of significant coronary disease.

Suppose a male patient has a negative stress test result but has multiple coronary risk factors. In this case the physician will wish to refine the diagnostic accuracy of the stress test with the thallium scan. This test has a higher degree of sensitivity and diagnostic accuracy and is used when the presence of significant disease is strongly suspected but the stress test has yielded a conflicting result.

On the other hand, a patient devoid of all risk factors who tests positive on the normal treadmill can also benefit from the more accurate thallium scan.

Stress testing is advised for any man above 35 who has the presence of at least one other significant cardiovascular risk factor. People in this category should be stress-tested annually. If a woman has multiple risk factors for CHD, she is treated as equivalent to her male counterpart.

Another value of the stress test is its ability to give your functional exercise capacity. Knowing the amount of aerobic expenditure you have put into a stress test can help your physician design an aerobic program specifically for your needs. Anyone above the age of 30 should consult with his or her physician about the need for stress testing prior to beginning a vigorous aerobic program.

### *Monitoring Your Heart Rate*

You will find a strong, vigorous carotid pulse present on both sides of your neck when you are exercising aerobically. All you have to do is count your heartbeat at the location of the carotid pulse for six seconds and multiply it by ten and you will have your heart rate in terms of the number of beats per minute. Do this on a daily basis before you begin exercising to get an idea just what your resting pulse is so that in a three-to-six-month period of time, depending upon the regularity of the aerobic exercise, you can monitor the deceleration of your pulse as a reflection of the adequacy of your aerobic exercise. Rapid deceleration of the heartbeat following vigorous aerobic exercise implies cardiovascular fitness. When you are cardiovascularly fit you should have a slow resting pulse. A slow resting pulse is, of course, relative. In a middle-aged person a slow resting pulse may be in the low 60s to mid 50s. Generally speaking, one should have a slow resting pulse, a pulse that accelerates gradually in response to aerobic stimulation, not rapidly.

If a person has a rapid resting pulse, a pulse that accelerates rapidly in response to aerobic activity, and a pulse that remains accelerated following aerobic exercise, that person probably has a deconditioned heart. If that is the case for you, as you monitor your heart and practice your aerobic activity regularly, you should note a gradual reversal in this pattern of deconditioning as you become more fit.

A slow heart rate in a person who practices regular, consistent aerobic exercise is good; a slow heart rate in an older person who is sedentary may be a very bad sign.

It is also advisable to monitor your pulse rate during exercise to avoid overstressing your heart muscle. Be sensitive to a too rapid heartbeat.

When you are exercising on a regular basis—at least three times a week for a period of half an hour or more—it is only necessary to push yourself to within 70 to 75 percent of the maximum heart rate for your age.

**Maximum Heart Rate By Age**

| *Age* | *Maximum Heart Rate* |
|---|---|
| 20 | 200 |
| 25 | 195 |
| 30 | 190 |
| 35 | 185 |
| 40 | 180 |
| 41 | 175 |
| 45 | 170 |
| 50 | 165 |
| 55 | 160 |
| 60 | 155 |
| 65 | 150 |
| 70 | 145 |
| 75 | 140 |
| 80 | 135 |

## *SETTING UP YOUR OWN AEROBIC PROGRAM*

Your ability to engage in a regular, vigorous aerobic program has to be verified by your physician before you begin the activity. If your lifestyle has been a relatively sedentary one, it is the repetition of the pattern that is more important than the duration of each exercise period. It is much better to start out for 5 minutes four times a week and gradually build up your stamina. Risk, dietary, and exercise modification are all a matter of the slow, gradual change and habituation that will bring about prolonged benefit.

When it comes to exercise, the important thing to realize is that it is best to start slowly. Repetition of brief periods of exercise in the beginning will enable you to advance to more prolonged periods of activity. Exercise is one of the last places you should attempt to seek instant gratification. To do so is dangerous. You do not have to build hefty muscles to be physically fit. If you like to swim, swim for at least 30 minutes three times a week. If you like to walk, walk 3 or 4 miles three times a week. If you like to ride a bicycle, ride a bike starting with 1 mile three times a week and as you become stronger, gradually increase the distance. Keep the goal in mind: It is not to win a marathon, it is not to have a muscular body—it is to live a long, productive, healthy life.

## *HDLS AND AEROBIC EXERCISE*

A reduced HDL cholesterol level puts you at an increased risk for CHD and is classified as a major risk factor. The major causes of reduced HDL levels are listed in the table on page 118. Heavy cigarette smoking reduces HDL levels. When it is accompanied by heavy drinking of coffee, the reduction is even greater. Hypertriglyceridemia is associated with reduced HDL, as is the use of anabolic steroids and progestational agents. Obesity is a major cause of reduced HDL levels. A lack of physical activity may also reduce your HDL levels. The regular practice of aerobic exercise may increase your HDLs.

## *WATCH YOUR DENIAL*

Psychological denial is a tool we all use at one time or another, but when it comes to managing your cholesterol you

| Fig. 11 Major Causes of Reduced Serum HDL-Cholesterol |
|---|
| Cigarette Smoking |
| Obesity |
| Lack of exercise |
| Androgenic and related steroids |
| Androgens |
| Progestational agents |
| Anabolic steroids |
| β-Adrenergic blocking agents |
| Hypertriglyceridemia |
| Genetic factors |
| Primary hypoalphalipoproteinemia |

will want to be aware of any tendency not to squarely face the facts in this life-or-death matter. Don't tell yourself you are getting adequate aerobic exercise when all of the evidence indicates that you are not. Do not tell yourself you are going to start exercising tomorrow when you know you have not made sufficient arrangements and adjustments to fit it into your routine. Exercise is an essential component to effective cholesterol management. On the other hand, do not deny the need to lose weight, to eat less, to eat more nutritionally, or to take your medication.

Doctors tend to find it extremely difficult to cope with the denial mechanism that many patients with asymptomatic diseases such as hypertension, diabetes, and elevated cholesterol have. It appears that people who do not feel the symptom are more apt to question "Why do I have to do this?" Beware of ignoring your dietary restrictions or your exercise program because you feel all right.

Do not deny the necessity of participating in your own health care. For example, patients who have total cholesterol in the 400 mg/dl range who consistently go off their diet and miss medication schedules manifest a far more severe degree of peripheral vascular disease and coronary disease at a much earlier age than do those who adhere to the program without denial.

> *In diabetes, hypertension, and elevated cholesterol, the acceleration of target organ damage is similar; all of these diseases affect the network of arteries in the brain, the heart, and the kidneys. The degree and severity of the damage these metabolic diseases inflict upon the target organs depends upon the lack of control of the disorder. All of these diseases are asymptomatic; you may feel good while vital organs are being irreversibly damaged.*
>
> —DR. ALAN BECKLES

## *MAKING LIFESTYLE ADJUSTMENTS*

Perhaps you travel a lot in your business and wonder how to get in regular aerobic exercise. You may practice yoga in your hotel room, run in place, or check the local TV schedule to see if there is an early morning aerobic dancing show. Choose hotel accommodations that include a health spa where you can swim or use the exercise room. If you prefer walking or running, ask at the reception desk for safe places to walk or run. One woman who travels a lot in her job always packs her jumping rope.

Make it a habit in advance of the trip to think about finding restaurants that are known for serving wholesome food in the place where you are going. Ask your travel agent, airlines, and hotel for information. You can often find telephone books and the Yellow Pages for most major cities at the library. Ask other people who have traveled to the area, or people you know who live there. If all else fails, as soon as you arrive secure a Yellow Pages where you will find many ads. Call the restaurants that appear to offer what you need and ask about menu items and food preparation.

In nearly every medium to large city in this country you

can find restaurants that are popular and not off the beaten track where a strong attempt is made to prepare food organically.

Suppose you don't have the opportunity to choose the restaurants you will be eating in. Select salads that are not laden with fat and cholesterol dressings made with bacon and egg yolk, shrimp, or ham. Fish prepared in the most nutritional fashion and a raw spinach salad without bacon and with alfalfa and bean sprouts make excellent choices. Since you are on a cholesterol-lowering diet, ask the chef to do you a special favor and prepare you a large mixed vegetable salad served with the lightest dressing. Lemon, vinegar, and oil with spices is an excellent choice. If this does not provide enough bulk for you, have a baked potato (without sour cream; use margarine) and a small piece of broiled fish or a very lean cut of beef.

Suppose your schedule is such that you really do not have time to eat breakfast. Keep an ample supply of your favorite pure juices available. Eat two pieces of fruit or drink a glass or two of pure fruit juice and start your day nutritionally.

Remember: Low fat, high fiber, and aerobic exercise are *pro* life!

# 6
# Your Child's Diet Is Important Too

The dietary needs of growing children until age 19 are different from those of adults. Children need lots of calcium, iron, and protein for healthy bones, teeth, hair, and muscles. Therefore, it is not advisable to restrict their intake of dairy products. The dietary restrictions that apply to adults cannot apply to growing children. In fact, dietary restrictions in children can result in poor bone growth and skeletal abnormalities. The American Academy of Pediatrics recommends a total fat intake for children of 30 to 40 percent of calories. The American Heart Association, on the other hand, recommends that children over 2 years old limit their fat intake to 30 percent of calories. Of course, you will want to keep a proper balance between saturated fats and unsaturated fats. You will also want to take care not to foster obesity in a young child.

The most important thing to do for your children is to establish dietary habits from birth that do not encourage them to eat fast foods, fried foods, junk foods, and sweets. You will want to encourage your children to avoid simple sugars and foods high in saturated fat. Use raw fruits and vegetables as snacks; make candy and ice cream rare treats. Limit the amount of chocolate your children ingest. There is very little nutritional value in candy, sugars, and chocolate. To restrict your child's intake of these items is beneficial without being harmful since they are not sources of calcium and protein.

It is well known that according to autopsy studies so-called blue streaks are found in the coronary arteries of small children and infants. Blue streaks are thought to represent the earliest atherosclerotic lesion in coronary arteries. Nevertheless, there is no reason to limit children's total fat/cholesterol intake below 30 percent. Children should be taught dietary habits they can carry into adulthood.

Generally speaking, as adults we stop growing and become increasingly sedentary. Our need for nutritional and caloric intake is not as great as that of a growing child. In many instances it is considerably less, but too often we continue eating at the same rate as we did when we were children.

When we enter adulthood and begin to realize that we will need to restrict our food intake, the good habits learned in childhood will lessen the need for severe modification. One woman tells of how her three school-age children complained bitterly because she refused to put Twinkies in their lunch boxes, giving them fruit instead. They were also upset because she made their sandwiches with whole grain bread and never used luncheon meats when all of their classmates had lunches made with Wonder bread and an assortment of cold cuts. Now that her children are in their twenties they thank their mother for helping them to avoid the sugar addiction they see in so many of their friends. They are also pleased to have healthy diets that need little adjustment as they lead disease-free, active lives.

Replace soda pop with naturally sweetened fruit juices. Bake or buy desserts sweetened with honey or brown sugar. Use sugar-free whole grain cereals such as granola or oatmeal and teach your child to lightly sweeten them with unprocessed honey. Encourage your child to eat healthy servings of whole grain cereals and fresh fruit for breakfast. Use whole wheat bread and naturally sweetened jams and jellies. Since you will want to discourage fried foods, teach your children while they are still very young to eat poached or boiled eggs for breakfast. The occasional fried egg can serve as a special treat. Use vegetable oil for frying. French fries are a favorite American fried food. Teach your children how to enjoy the potato in more wholesome forms, saving french fries for a special treat.

Obesity in your child can lead to early development of atherosclerosis. Additionally, it usually places the child at a psychological disadvantage in a society that places much emphasis on slimness. Encourage eating habits that discourage obesity.

Teach your children to live and play in ways that guarantee plenty of aerobic exercise. Encourage your boys and girls to choose an activity such as biking, hiking, or skating early in life so that they can carry the practice of it right into adulthood. Teach children from the beginning that adequate exercise is necessary at all ages. Too many active people become sedentary as soon as they reach adulthood. Good physical habits are as important as good eating habits.

Keep in mind that heart disease develops for years and years without any sign.

Children who have a severely elevated cholesterol for genetic reasons— who are homozygous because of a recessive gene that determines LDL number and function and are unable to produce LDL receptors in sufficient number, or adequately functioning ones—will need dietary restrictions similar to those outlined in the Step One Diet. If not placed on such a diet, they may suffer a premature heart attack in their 20s.

Some children are the victims of Tangiers disease, a rare genetic disorder in which HDL is completely absent. These victims suffer from severe elevations in serum cholesterol, and dietary restrictions have to be instituted to avoid the possibility of a heart attack in their 20s.

A good physical examination and ordinary laboratory screening ought to reveal any child who has severely elevated serum cholesterol totals. Severe genetic predispositions to cholesterol elevation should be picked up very early in a child's life.

Barring the rare occurrence of genetically induced high cholesterol levels, good dietary habits established as early as possible in your child's life will assure good health.

You will want to ascertain that your child consumes a healthy, wholesome, balanced diet. If red meat is included in your child's diet, you will want to make sure that it is lean. You will want to watch the environmental influences on your child to guarantee that he or she doesn't pick up negative nutritional cues. Give your children's birthday parties at home where you can prepare and serve wholesome, tasty food. If you want, you can hire a clown or a juggler to come and entertain the children. There are many creative, fun alternatives to a fast-food party for your child and his or her playmates.

If you are nutritionally aware as a parent, you will begin to restrict outside influences that offer your children negative nutritional cues. You will need to encourage relatives and friends not to give your children food that you do not approve of. If your children are going to visit a friend or relative who has very relaxed dietary standards, pack a lunch for them and ask that they be fed the food you have sent along with them at mealtime. Be firm and specific about the things you do or do not want your children to eat. Tell them and tell those in whose company they will be exactly what your dietary expectations are. Ask friends and relatives not to give your children hot dogs as a treat, not to give them hamburgers as a treat—most especially not to give them simple sugars (candy, ice cream, and baked goods) as a treat. Give anyone, baby-sitters and grandparents included, strict instructions about what your child is to be fed either as a full meal or as a snack. Do not leave the development of your child's dietary habits to others and to chance!

By finding wholesome alternatives, you can raise a child who as an adult does not crave sweets, sodas, potato chips, and fried foods excessively. It really is a matter of discipline and the willingness to make the extra effort to give your child a better start in life. Most parents want the very best for their children. Diet and nutrition should be no exception. Just as you insist on good work in school, make sure your children eat what is good for them.

Children's dietary habits and exercise habits are programmed relatively early in life. It is very important once the child begins to take solid food on a regular basis that the parents make a sincere effort so the child will not develop poor dietary habits that in adulthood can lead to premature disease. It will be important for parents to practice good dietary habits themselves before their children. Good eating is a family affair.

Involve your young children in activities that guarantee enough exercise. Develop habits and tastes that will promote a lifetime of adequate exercise. If you carry out appropriate exercises before your child, as soon as that child develops sufficient motor coordination to begin to do simple exercises he or she will do them out of pure imitation. We set the pattern very early for the type of lifestyle our children will most likely choose. Current patterns encourage a very high incidence of premature death by heart attack.

Help your children learn to eat fresh, whole foods that are

low in saturated fat and high in nutritional value. Encourage them to satisfy cravings for sweets with fruit, and most especially teach them early to avoid fried and highly processed foods.

Keeping your blood lipids in a healthy balance is a lifelong effort. Help your children to establish the right habits now.

## *GLOSSARY*

**Aduki beans:** Also spelt as *adzuki* or adsuki is edible brown seeds widely cultivated in Japan and China. In Japanese adzuki means red-beans.

**Angel food cake:** Very light sponge cake.

**Asparagus:** *Shatwari, soot mooli.*

**Black-eyed peas:** Rongi, lobhia.

**Brisket:** Breast meat.

**Broccoli:** A variety of cauliflower.

**Caviar:** Pickled small deer.

**Chicken cacciatore:** Continental dish made with chicken, tomato, brown sauce, mushroom, rosemary herb and red wine.

**Chuck:** Neck and shoulder meat.

**Collard:** A smooth-leaved variety of kale.

**Corned:** Preserved or tinned meat.

**Coleslaw:** Salad made of raw, sliced cabbage leaves.

**Cranapples:** A variety of cranberries *(vaccinium),* also called edible red barries.

**Croissants:** A variety of bread roll.

**Crudite salad:** To have vegetable salad dipped in sauce.

**Dandelion:** Lion's tooth.

**Eggnog:** Solanum melongena, aubergine.

**Escarole:** Endive plant leaves.

**Flank:** Fleshy part between the ribs and the hips.

**French fries:** Potato chips.

**Frosting:** Icing.

**Gazpacho:** Spanish cold vegetable soup.

**Graham crackers:** Crackers made of flour.

**Granola:** A preparation made of ground cereals rich in wheat, corn etc. A sort of dalia.

**Halibut:** *Amriki malli*

**Jalapeno cornbread:** Jalapeno is Maxican chilli; hence cornbread mixed with Maxican chilli.

**Linguine:** A variety of pasta.

**Lunch meat:** Meat in loaf form.

**Matzo:** A kind of bread.

**Melba toast:** Thin crisp toast.

**Muffin:** Small bread cake eaten with butter.

**Mung beans:** The edible green yellow seeds of an errect bushy annual bean *(Phaseolus aureus)*—widely cultivated in warm region.

**Navy beans:** A white dried bean—so called from its use by the US Navy.

**Picante sauce:** Sauce made with spices.

**Pintos:** A variety of kidney beans from southwest US.

**Pita bread:** Bread made from fibre yielding plants such as pineapple, agave or yucca in Spain and Portugal.

**Pretzels:** A crisp, glazed, salted, knot-shaped cracker.

**Pumpernickel bread:** Brown bread.

**Ratatouille:** Provincial stew of vegetables.

**Saltines:** A crisp, thin, salted cracker.

**Spinach fettuccine:** A variety of pasta.

**Swiss chard:** A kind of beat.

**T-bone:** Fleshy part from loin.

**Tofu or tofu recipes:** Cheese made of soya milk.

**Tortilla chips:** Thin flat maize cake.

**Tuna:** *Valaiti bangra.*

**Vichyssoise:** Creamy soup of leeks and potatoes.

**Waffles:** Small crisp cake.

**Zucchini:** Small variety of vegetable marrow.